Economics and
Medical Research

Economics and
Medical Research

Burton A. Weisbrod

American Enterprise Institute for Public Policy Research
Washington and London

Library of Congress Cataloging in Publication Data

Weisbrod, Burton Allen, 1931–
    Economics and medical research.

    (AEI studies; 373)
    Includes bibliographical references.
    1. Medical research—Economic aspects—United
States. 2. Medical research—United States—Cost
effectiveness. 3. Medical care—United States—
Cost effectiveness. 4. Medical research—Economic
aspects—United States—Case studies. 5. Medical
research—United States—Cost effectiveness—Case
studies. 6. Medical care—United States—Cost
effectiveness—Case studies. I. Title. II. Series.
R854.U5W4   1983   338.4'761'072073   82–22819

ISBN 0–8447–3513–2
ISBN 0–8447–3512–4 (pbk.)

AEI Studies 373

 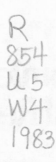
Printed in the United States of America

Contents

LIST OF TABLES

LIST OF FIGURES

Preface

This volume focuses on medical research and its effects on the health care system. Medical research and medical technology are typically discussed as if they were affected primarily by noneconomic factors. Government grants, through the National Institutes of Health (NIH), dominate basic research on health. Research by profit-making firms—such as those in the pharmaceutical industry—is related to expected profitability, but the research financed by government and private nonprofit organizations is seldom analyzed in terms of its costs and benefits.

There are two sets of issues. One is normative, policy-oriented: What proportion of our resources should be allocated to medical research? What lines of research should be pursued? At what speed? How should "basic" and "applied" research be balanced? How should society allocate research resources between diseases affecting older people and diseases affecting youngsters? How should the importance of research on reducing pain—for example, from such diseases as arthritis—be compared with the importance of research on reducing mortality? This raises questions about how to "value" reduction in pain and increases in life expectancy. When mental illness is considered, the scope of normative issues becomes even broader. Although mental illness sometimes contributes to premature mortality, it typically affects not longevity but the ability to cope with life's problems and, hence, the quality of life.

The second set of issues is positive: how are decisions made about the types of medical research to support, and at what levels? What values are placed—implicitly or explicitly—by private and public decision makers on the importance of increased understanding of the causes of and cures for various diseases? On the relative importance of extending life and reducing pain? On the relative importance of basic and applied research? How do technical advances resulting from research influence the accessibility of medical care to persons with low income? How does medical research affect the health insurance market? Reciprocally, how does health insurance affect the course of medical research?

Our severely limited understanding of decision-making processes in medical research reflects the deeper inadequacy of knowledge about goals, constraints, and decision processes in the institutions that dominate the health industry—government and private nonprofit organizations. Since most basic medical research is financed by the federal government—60 percent in 1980[1]—and much of that is spent at private nonprofit universities and other nonprofit institutions, it is clear that to understand and predict how resources are allocated to medical research, we must learn more about the behavior of these nonproprietary institutions. If proprietary firms are profit maximizers, subject to the constraints of market demand, market prices of input resources, and the state of technology, how should government institutions and private nonprofit organizations be characterized and modeled? Indeed, is there a single way of describing the "objective functions" (goals) of all government organizations and the constraints on them—from regulatory agencies such as the Food and Drug Administration (FDA) and the Occupational Safety and Health Administration (OSHA), to operating agencies such as NIH, to the judiciary, legislatures, and others? Is it possible to develop a single model of the behavior of such varied entities as nonprofit hospitals, nursing homes, medical research organizations (for muscular dystrophy, epilepsy, and so on), and organizations devoted to training or providing income to the mentally and physically handicapped?

The need for improved models to predict the behavior of all governmental and private nonproprietary organizations is considerable, but nowhere is it greater than in the health area, where these forms of institutions are dominant: (1) Most basic medical research is financed by one sector, government; it is performed by another, private nonprofit universities; and the results are implemented by a third sector, proprietary firms. (2) Nonprofit organizations provide the majority of short-stay hospital beds, 64 percent in 1979.[2] (3) Government finances a growing proportion of personal medical care expenditures, from 21.8 percent in 1960 to 39.6 percent in 1980.[3] (4) Private nonprofit insurers, particularly Blue Cross and Blue Shield, serve 47 percent of the population.[4]

The role of nonproprietary organizations in medical research, medical care, and health insurance suggests strongly that the health sector is atypical of our predominantly private-market economy. Medical care—its production, distribution, and financing—is indeed different. But in what sense is it different? How should the differences affect the way society identifies problems in the medical care area, and how should they affect the social policies through which society attempts to deal with the problems?

The following chapters only scratch the surface of answers to these questions. After an introductory chapter that expands on the issues touched on here and another that takes up the question whether medical care really is different from other services and industries (chapter 2), the subsequent chapters of part 1 direct attention to the methods and problems of evaluating medical care programs in both physical and mental health (chapters 3 and 4). The case studies in part 2 apply benefit-cost analysis to three quite different innovations— a vaccine against poliomyelitis (chapter 5), a complex set of techniques for treating the mentally ill (chapter 6), and a new therapeutic drug for control of duodenal ulcers (chapter 7).

These studies illustrate both the potential for, and the limitations of, quantitative evaluation in the medical care area. I hope they will stimulate further efforts to assess the fruits of medical research. Each of the three innovations evaluated in part 2 is a recent addition to the arsenal of treatment technologies. The economic consequences of medical research, which lead to such new technologies, are the real focus of this book. More attention is badly needed to the ramifications of a multibillion-dollar annual medical research program that combines profit-making firms, nonprofit charities (American Cancer Society), government grants and intramural research (NIH), and nonprofit performance of research (universities) and that interacts in complex ways with the entire medical care market. That market creates incentives that affect the direction and profitability of medical research and the level of expenditures on medical care (this interaction is examined in chapter 3). While much has been written about the economics of medical insurance, there has been scant attention to the economics of medical research and still less to the interplay of insurance and research.

My hope is that this set of papers will be useful to several audiences—to students and scholars interested in the economics of health, to researchers contemplating benefit-cost analyses or other studies dealing with health care and medical research and development, and to all who wish to see how one economist views the medical research and health care markets and the opportunities for benefit-cost evaluation of the technical innovations they generate.

Most of this book consists of revisions or reprintings of my previously published work. Chapter 1, however, an overview of issues, and the concluding chapter were written for this volume.

Notes

1. U.S. Department of Health and Human Services, *Health—United States* (Washington, D.C., 1981), p. 215.
2. Ibid., p. 251.
3. Ibid., p. 770.
4. *Source Book of Health Insurance Data, 1981–1982* (Washington, D.C.: Health Insurance Association of America, 1982), p. 13.

Acknowledgments

I thank the following publishers for permitting me to include previously published works: Aspen Systems Corporation, Almqvist and Wiksell Company, National Institute of Mental Health, Hoffmann-LaRoche, Inc., *The Journal of Political Economy* (University of Chicago Press), *The Journal of Human Resources* (University of Wisconsin Press), Academic Press, and the American Enterprise Institute for Public Policy Research.

I also thank my collaborators, who agreed to publication of our joint papers in this volume—John Geweke, John Goddeeris, Thomas McGuire, and Mark Schlesinger. Felicity Skidmore edited an earlier version of the manuscript and made valuable suggestions for its revision.

Finally, I thank Robert Helms, who originally suggested this volume when he was director of health policy studies at the American Enterprise Institute. He proposed that I put together a number of my published papers that dealt with health issues in general, and medical research in particular. I agreed with the idea, but with reservations. Whatever my contributions may have been, they are but a portion of the economics literature dealing with benefit-cost analysis and the assessment of medical research and technological change in the health and medical care area.

PART ONE

Issues in the Evaluation of Health Care

1

An Economic Perspective on Medical Research

This chapter examines the role of medical research within the larger economic-political context and considers the forces affecting the amount, direction, and consequences of such research. Economists have been concerned with the appropriate role of scientific research for decades, even centuries. Yet the attention they have given to the economic role and consequences of medical research has been minuscule. There has been a scarcity of quantitative information and of knowledge about qualitative relationships. This essay points toward the need for further research; at the same time it provides background for the chapters that follow.

This chapter is an overview of issues relating to medical research and its causes and consequences, from an economic perspective. The principal topics discussed are the influence of the private nonprofit sector in the provision of funds for medical research; the effects of successful medical research on the demand for health-care insurance and, reciprocally, the effects of insurance on the level and direction of medical research; the relationship between the rising expenditures on medical care and social welfare; the problem of measuring benefits from improved health; the consequences of consumer ignorance in determining the productivity (quality and value) of health services; some unusual aspects of measuring productivity of mental health services; and the problem of how to choose among health programs when different but well-identified population groups are affected.

Since economists have paid scant attention to the nonprofit sector in any context, it is not surprising that the medical research funded or performed by this sector has been neglected.[1] Research on the economics of government, though substantial overall, has also directed little specific attention to the medical research budget—how it is determined, how it should be determined, and what its effects are. Yet since 1965, research and development expenditures of the National Institutes of Health alone grew from $595 million (4 percent of total federal spending for research and development) to $1.7 billion by 1975 (8.6 percent), and to an estimated $3.6 billion by 1982 (9.3 percent).[2] The long-term consequences of medical research may well be enormous; according to one recent estimate, 30 to 40 percent of the reduction in deaths in the United States between 1900 and 1975 is accounted for by biomedical advance.[3]

It is no coincidence that the growth of medical research and development expenditures has been accompanied by the growth, indeed the surge, of private and governmental programs to insure patients against the high costs of medical care. The purpose of private health insurance and such governmental programs as Medicare and Medicaid has been to improve financial access to high-quality medical care, but the effects have been broader. Private and public insurance have increased the amount of marginally useful, unproductive, and even counterproductive surgery and other therapy. It has pushed up physicians' incomes. It has spurred the development of a proprietary hospital industry. But what has been its effect on the rate and direction of medical research? This important question has only recently begun to be examined.[4]

One effect of health insurance (of the types currently available) is to provide a ready market for medical innovations. In the short run the marginal cost to a patient is no different whether the treatment uses an older technology or one that is newer and slightly more effective, but considerably more costly.[5] Not only patients but also medical-care providers and entrepreneurs have less incentive to hold down costs, or to search for or develop lower-cost technologies than they would have without such insurance.

It is no accident that the soaring political pressures for expanded health insurance have come on the heels of unprecedented breakthroughs in medical research. As medical research alters the state of knowledge about the prevention, treatment, and cure of illness, it also affects the demand for insurance. Only decades ago medicine was capable of doing relatively little for an afflicted person. Illness, even terminal illness, did not lead to large medical care expenditures because the state of knowledge did not permit it. As a result, there was little demand—in either a market or a political sense—for health insurance.

The advances of modern medicine have changed all that. No longer need kidney disease lead to quick death; with small medical expenditures on the part of the patient, effective but extremely costly kidney dialysis is available. Advances in artificial resuscitation techniques are preventing many deaths from drowning, but sometimes with the result of costly and protracted maintenance of severely brain-

4

FIGURE 1-1

THE MEDICAL RESEARCH CIRCLE

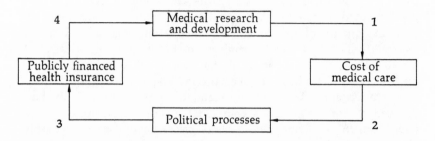

damaged people. Advances in research on artificial organs have produced a workable artificial heart and, soon, an artificial lung but with staggering cost implications.[6]

It is difficult to know how much of the growth in medical care expenditures can be attributed to more widespread and comprehensive insurance coverage. Whatever the answer may be, however, the question will remain: Why has health insurance expanded so rapidly? After all, the demand for insurance is not a random matter determined by chance factors.

The explanation for the growth of health insurance as a result of medical "success," discussed in chapter 3, follows these lines: (1) successful medical research has led to new therapies that are effective but more costly than previously existing technology; (2) these new opportunities have sometimes confronted individuals with life-and-death choices that are made difficult because of their high cost; (3) the financial stress has manifested itself in political pressure to provide access for all citizens to the new health-care opportunities; (4) this pressure has encouraged the government to increase its financing of health care—directly through Medicare and Medicaid or indirectly by making employee-financed health insurance tax deductible and employer-financed health insurance nontaxable to the employee; and (5) the growing availability of health insurance has blunted the sensitivity of consumers and health-care providers to the costliness of new technologies and thereby affected the forms and directions of medical research and development. Thus the causal circle is closed, as shown in figure 1-1. The rising national expenditures on medical care, the growth of health-care insurance, and the forms of medical research are all parts of an interdependent system.

There is an important distinction to be made in the use of terms. To equate health-care expenditures with health-care costs is common

5

but misleading and confuses the forces that are at work. Expenditures have soared in significant part because the quality of health-care technology has improved dramatically. But it is only partially true that costs are now higher for obtaining the same type of care today that was provided yesterday. A hospital is not what it is was formerly: even the quality of its "hotel" accommodations has improved dramatically. Two-bed rooms, semiprivate bathrooms, electrically adjustable beds, color television, better meals, and a host of standby medical capabilities have replaced the more spartan hospital ward of a generation ago. As our living standards have improved, we have demanded more from the accommodations of our hospitals as we have from those of our hotels, where prices have also risen sharply. This suggests that more is responsible for the growing expenditures than the interplay of medical research and health care insurance. Sorting out the separate influences and their interdependencies is yet another area calling for more knowledge.

Budget and cost-cutting considerations have shaped not only the political debate but also the character of much economic research, with the result that costs have been studied far more exhaustively than benefits. This is understandable because governmental financial support is available for economic research on costs—usually for the purpose of controlling expenditures—and data on costs are easier to obtain. Yet efficient resource allocation requires attention to benefits as well as costs.

The dearth of economic research on benefits from the knowledge generated by medical research is striking. Increased expenditures on any commodity, health care or other, do not necessarily represent either an increase or a decrease in welfare. In typical economic-theoretic models, involving assumptions of well-informed consumers and competitive producers, an increase in expenditures signals an improvement in welfare when demand increases in response to an increase in quality. Why, then, does so much of the policy debate rest on the assumption that the rising expenditures on medical care represent a decrease in welfare? One answer is the belief that insurance has distorted decisions by not confronting consumers and providers with the full social consequences of their actions. Yet it is not clear that this is anywhere near the full answer.

What are the benefits from medical research, how can they be measured, and how should they be valued for comparison with social costs? To answer these questions, the effect of research on mortality and life expectancy is often examined. The considerable literature on this subject, however, has generally not come to grips with certain

TABLE 1-1

Costs per Death Averted, 1968–1972

(dollars)

Program	Program Cost per Death Averted
Seat-belt use	87
Motorcycle helmets	3,336
Uterine cervix cancer	3,470
Lung cancer	6,400
Syphilis	22,252
Colon-rectum cancer	42,944
Arthritis	n.a.

Note: n.a. = not applicable.
Source: U.S. Department of Health, Education, and Welfare, *Selected Disease Control Programs*, September 1966, p. 34.

fundamental weaknesses in the use of mortality rates and life expectancy as measures of welfare.[7]

1. Morbidity and quality of life are dimensions of welfare not captured by, and often not even correlated positively with, changes in mortality. Arthritis, for example, causes much discomfort, pain, and disruption of normal life, but has little direct effect on mortality. Thus, the U.S. Department of Health, Education, and Welfare was unable to deal with arthritis in a statistical analysis of "costs per death averted" from a variety of antidisease programs, as shown in table 1-1.

2. Table 1-1 illustrates another common deficiency of evaluations of health programs (including medical research) that focus on mortality or, in this case, on "deaths averted." Just as one cannot tell whether a death averted means that the person lived a normal life or an extremely restricted one, so such statistics say nothing about how much longer the person lived. Medical research that averts death may postpone the inevitable for a long time or for only a short period. Data on life expectancy would reveal the distinction, but data on deaths averted do not. And, as noted above, the quality of life possible for the persons whose deaths were averted could range from a full life to that of a "vegetable" and is in no way captured by either mortality or life-expectancy data alone.

3. In considering the effect of medical research on longevity or morbidity, an important conceptual question is often overlooked:

What should be the basis for comparison, the basis for defining the counterfactual? Should comparisons be based on some measure of health status, say, life expectancy, (a) before and after some advance in medical research, or (b) with and without that advance, other things equal, or (c) with and without the advance, allowing for changes in behavior as a result of the new technology?

It does make a difference. The shortcomings of the before-after as compared with the with-without conceptual experiment are well known, but the choice between (b) and (c) is more involved. Medical research may well bring forth an innovation that would improve health status if the behavior of people were not otherwise altered. If, however, the innovation caused a change in behavior as people, now less fearful of certain consequences, adjusted their life styles, then we might actually observe little or no improvement in the measure of health status. Examples of such results from an innovation abound, both outside and within the health area. Better brakes on automobiles may lead to faster driving and more, not fewer, accidents, even though the improved brakes would clearly reduce accidents if behavior—in this case, speeding—had not changed. A flood control dam may well lead to an expansion of capital investment on a flood plain and thus to more, not less, injury and flood damage, even though the dam would clearly reduce damage if investment behavior had not changed. Improved health resulting from medical research may lead to increased desire for vacation time and thus to more, not less, on-the-job absenteeism, even though the improved health status would clearly have reduced absenteeism if attitudes toward leisure had not changed. Discovery of the effectiveness of antibiotics in treating certain venereal diseases may lead to an increase, not a decrease, in venereal diseases as sexual activity increases in response to the reduced danger, even though the discovery would clearly have reduced the prevalence and incidence of these diseases if sexual behavior had not changed.

There are two important lessons in these illustrations. One is that it is all too easy to use measures of health care benefits that, though plausible, actually give erroneous indications; gauging the benefits from research on automobile brakes by accident rates, on dam construction by flood damage, and on antibiotics by venereal disease rates will systematically understate the full benefits, possibly even seem to show negative benefits. The second lesson—another aspect of the first—is that while most people want improved health, they also want other things, and they are willing to give up some health benefits in exchange. As a result, the total benefits from medical research include not only those that are manifest in improved health but also others that appear in a wide variety of options open to persons willing to take their expanded opportunities in other forms.

The question of how to value benefits from medical research—once the forms of benefits have been identified—is a critical issue. Economists have given much attention to questions of the value of human life, of the alleviation of pain and suffering, and of other dimensions of the quality of life. But the issues remain controversial. To some economists, especially during the 1960s, it has seemed useful to think in terms of human capital, that is, the market value of a person as a productive labor asset (see chapter 5 for one example). More recently conventional economic analysis has used the willingness-to-pay approach, in which the value of anything that affects individuals' utility—improved health being viewed as just such a commodity—is defined by willingness (and ability) to pay for it.[8]

Whatever its appeal to economists, willingness to pay is, to many others, an ambiguous, or even irrelevant, conceptual basis for placing a value on health and medical care.[9] First, it can make a great deal of difference whether one attempts to estimate the sum that people will pay for some health input or the sum they would require to be paid to them to forgo receiving that input (the "compensating variation" versus the "equivalent variation"). Second, either of these notions highlights the fact that economic demand depends on the distribution of money income, and it is a matter of considerable ethical controversy how much, if at all, the availability of health resources to any person should depend on his or her income. Is health a special good such that access to it should not be rationed by market forces? This is an important ethical issue, and while economics can analyze the consequences of alternative rationing mechanisms, it cannot determine their wisdom.

A recent study highlights the importance of the life-valuation issue, although in the end it does not confront it. The study examined the cost of vaccinating people against pneumococcal pneumonia, and the effect of the vaccinations on (quality-adjusted) life expectancy at various ages.[10] More important than the findings about the level of costs is the pattern of cost per year of (quality-adjusted) life expectancy for persons at various ages. As figure 1–2 shows, the cost of extending life is far higher for young children than for senior citizens; the reason is essentially the far lower probability of death from pneumococcal pneumonia for youngsters. Is it "worth" $1,000 of resources to extend one person's life expectancy for one year—this being the cost for a program focusing on persons over sixty-five? (I disregard, for the present purpose, the quality-adjustment process.) If so, is it worth $6,000? $77,000? The question of where to draw

FIGURE 1–2

Cost of Pneumococcal Pneumonia Vaccination per Quality-Adjusted Life Year, by Age of Person

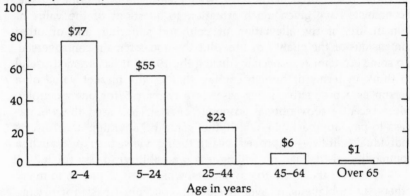

Cost per quality-adjusted life year ($000)

NOTE: The paper from which this is adapted explains the concept of a "quality-adjusted life year"; the basic notion is that a year of restricted mobility is "equivalent" to less than a year of "normal" life.
SOURCE: Adapted from Jane S. Willems et al., "Cost Effectiveness of Vaccination against Pneumococcal Pneumonia," *New England Journal of Medicine*, vol. 303 (September 14, 1980), p. 555.

the "line" is a question of how to value added longevity. It is also a question of how to assess the worth of medical research; if society is willing to incur costs of applying the fruits of research—in this case the vaccine—then the research has brought benefits. But if a social judgment were made that the cost of the vaccinations is "excessive" for everyone—to take an extreme example—we might conclude that the research that brought forth the vaccine was of no value, at least currently. In short, the value of research findings is inexorably entwined with the cost of applying those findings.

The literature on the effects of medical research has generally focused on the individual whose health status in such areas as life expectancy or disability has been improved. There are, however, macroeconomic effects from the extension of life expectancy, the extension of healthful (potential working) life expectancy, and the extension of retired-life expectancy. Changes in the age distribution of the population, for example—partially a result of advances in medical research—are already straining the social security budget. Growth in total population—again partially a consequence of advances in medical research—has brought growing pressure on the supply of land and other natural resources, such as fossil energy sources and national parks. Such effects are not examined in the benefit-cost analyses in chapters 5 through 7, but a full assessment of medical research policy would encompass effects that extend beyond health consequences.

Benefits from medical research are not limited to the country that pursues the research. Because the knowledge produced has the character of a collective good, it is available, despite some patent restrictions, throughout the world. But analysts, in restricting their attention to the United States, omit such international benefits, however substantial they may be.

Often the focus is narrowed still further: social benefits and costs are represented by flows of money to and from government. Clearly, however, there may be social benefits or costs without flows of money, and, conversely, there may be flows of money without real benefits or costs. (This is a major theme of the benefit-cost analysis in chapter 6.)

As a commodity, health care is by no means unique. But it is part of an unusual class of goods that is attracting growing attention. These are goods about the quality or effectiveness of which one party to a transaction is systematically better informed than the other party. The consumer of many health services—such as physician services, hospital or nursing home facilities, and pharmaceuticals—is generally ill-trained to judge their efficacy and quality. The providers, though also imperfectly informed, are usually more knowledgeable. This "informational asymmetry" characterizes not only much of the health care market but also, for example, legal representation, education, corporate "insider" transactions, and the used-car market and poses both efficiency and equity problems for decentralized private markets.[11] It is understandable that government has responded to this informational inequality by becoming involved as a regulator and a provider in the health care market, as in other markets. Whether the involvement is efficient, equitable, or justifiable, however, is another matter.

If consumers faced an unchanging product market, the passage of time and with it the experience of repeated purchases and information transfer would narrow the informational gap. If, however, the industry were characterized by rapid product change, infrequent purchase, and nonstandardized outputs, the informational asymmetry might well persevere. Such conditions—especially rapid technological change—have characterized the health industry in recent decades, as both privately and publicly financed research and development have brought forth a vast array of new drugs, surgical techniques, artificial organs, and other new technology and with them new institutional arrangements for providing and financing medical care. Informational problems abound and persist.

To cope with these informational problems, consumers rely on a number of mechanisms, such as agents (usually physicians), government regulation (of physicians, hospitals, and pharmaceutical firms, for example), and professional ethics codes. There has been little economic research, however, on the benefits, costs, and effectiveness of such mechanisms, generally and for particular subgroups of the population.[12]

Informational problems are nowhere more important than in the area of mental health. It is difficult to determine what constitutes an "improvement" in mental health and how to measure it. Yet without such a measure one cannot assess the productivity of any mental health resource, let alone compare the productivity, benefits, or cost effectiveness of various preventive or therapeutic measures (see chapters 2 and 6).

These difficulties have important implications. The inability to gauge the effectiveness of alternative inputs—let alone to value them—has contributed to the development of an ever-growing array of therapeutic resources that go beyond hospitals, physicians, nurses, psychiatric social workers, and drugs to include many types of community-based mechanisms such as halfway houses (see chapter 6) and group and individual measures such as transcendental meditation, transactional analysis, and "est." Work is now proceeding under the auspices of the National Institute of Mental Health (NIMH) on randomized controlled experiments to determine the effectiveness of various therapies.

Another implication of the difficulty of measuring productivity (and especially value added) is that health insurers face virtually limitless claims for mental health treatment costs and therefore tend to restrict, rather arbitrarily, the claims they will accept. The likelihood—indeed, the experience—that extremely high claims result when such constraints are absent arises from several factors: (1) Providers of mental health services can claim, with some justification, to be more knowledgeable than their patients about the effectiveness of the therapy; this is another illustration of informational asymmetry, as is the following point. (2) Insurers face an adverse-selection problem, the persons who most want mental health therapy being likely to gravitate toward insurance policies that are generous in their coverage for such therapy. (3) For some persons, seeing a mental health therapist is an expression not of illness in the usual rather vaguely defined sense but of loneliness—the desire to find someone to be with; the low, or even zero, marginal private cost to the patient encourages consumption even though alternatives exist that have lower social costs.

In public policy debates on national health insurance and in related scholarly research by economists, there has been remarkably little attention given to mental health costs. Yet the need for such attention is surely growing, as more of the population comes to accept mental illness as treatable and nonstigmatizing. Some of the issues are considered in chapters 4 and 6, below.[13]

There is sufficient reason to question the economic efficiency of the medical care market, given its characteristics. Medical care is an unusual commodity in that consumer evaluations are often suspect; health insurance and provider-compensation arrangements that distort incentives to acquire and use new technology are prevalent; and both governmental and private nonprofit organizations are substantially involved. Does the fact that so much of the health care industry is outside of profit-oriented organizations affect the rate of adoption of new medical technology and, in the process, affect the pace and direction of medical research? Assertions about "technological imperatives" aside, we have much to learn about how the institutional ownership of the health care industry affects and is affected by the medical research process.[14]

Evaluation of medical research and the medical care to which it is linked cannot proceed very far without confronting choices about the relative benefits of enhancing health for various identifiable population groups. Medical research decisions are seldom made from behind a Rawlsian "veil of ignorance"; that is, except at the most basic levels of research, we know that success in a particular line of research will tend to benefit, at least in the short run, one group or another—young people (polio vaccine research), middle-aged people (antiulcer drug research), the elderly (cancer research), women (cervical cancer research), men (prostate disease research), Jews (Tay-Sachs disease), those with kidney disease (research on renal dialysis), blacks (sickle-cell anemia), and so on. There is no way to be neutral.

Economic analysis alone can never determine policy decisions on the amount of resources to allocate to medical research or on the allocation of those resources among alternative research programs. Benefit-cost analysis, in particular, cannot determine finally whether a particular medical innovation is or is not efficient, let alone whether it is "desirable" in some larger social-welfare context. Nonetheless, benefit-cost analysis can help substantially to inform policy debate—to narrow the range of issues on which debate should focus.

I turn now to a series of examinations of some important aspects of health care markets. Following them, in part 2, are case studies that evaluate three areas of recent innovation in medical technology—the prevention or treatment of poliomyelitis, mental illness, and ulcers.

Notes

1. Three recent works on the private nonprofit sector are Burton A. Weisbrod, *The Voluntary Nonprofit Sector* (Lexington, Mass.: Lexington Books, 1977); Henry Hansmann, "The Role of Nonprofit Enterprise," *Yale Law Journal*, vol. 89 (1980): 835-901; and Michelle White, ed., *Nonprofit Firms in a Three Sector Economy* (Washington, D.C.: The Urban Institute, 1981).

2. National Science Foundation, *Federal Funds for Research and Development*, vol. 30, pp. 14, 16; vol. 25, pp. 4, 15; and vol. 15, pp. 4, 80.

3. Selma J. Mushkin, *Biomedical Research: Costs and Benefits* (Cambridge, Mass.: Ballinger Press, 1979), p. 5.

4. John Goddeeris, "Insurance, Technology and Medical Expenditures: A Study of Interactions," Ph.D. diss., Department of Economics, University of Wisconsin-Madison, 1980.

5. I refer to the effect of the "existing" type of insurance because the incentive structure would be different if insurance were of another type—in which insurance covered only care provided by a stipulated technology rather than by whatever technology was available.

6. Joan Arehart-Treichel, "An Artificial Heart in Search of a Patient," *Science News*, vol. 119 (March 7, 1981), p. 157; Lisa Nelson, "Implantable Artificial Lung Is Coming Closer to Reality, Brown University Researchers Say," *Wall Street Journal*, August 4, 1982.

7. Mushkin, *Biomedical Research*; John B. McKinlay and Sonja M. McKinlay, "The Questionable Contribution of Medical Research to the Decline of Mortality in the United States in the Twentieth Century," *Health and Society* (Milbank Memorial Fund Quarterly), vol. 55 (Summer 1977), pp. 405-428; Milton M. Chen and Douglas P. Wagner, "Gains in Mortality from Biomedical Research, 1930–1975: An Initial Assessment," *Social Science and Medicine*, vol. 12 (1978), pp. 73-81; and Solomon Schneyer, J. Steven Landefeld, and Frank H. Sandifer, "Biomedical Research and Illness: 1900–1979," *Health and Society* (Milbank Memorial Fund Quarterly), vol. 59 (1981), pp. 44-58. For consideration of quality of life, however, see Richard Zeckhauser and Donald Shepard, "Where Now for Saving Lives?" *Law and Contemporary Problems*, vol. 40 (1976), pp. 5-45.

8. For further discussion of issues in the valuation of life, see Ezra J. Mishan, "Evaluation of Life and Limb: A Theoretical Approach," *Journal of Political Economy*, vol. 19 (1971), pp. 687-705; Michael W. Jones-Lee, *The Value of Life: An Economic Analysis* (Chicago: University of Chicago Press, 1976); Richard Thaler and Sherwin Rosen, "Estimating the Value of a Life: Evidence from the Labor Market," in Nestor E. Terleckyj, ed., *House-*

hold *Production and Consumption* (New York: Columbia University Press, 1976); Zeckhauser and Shepard, "Where Now for Saving Lives?"

9. Steven Kelman, "Cost-Benefit Analysis: An Ethical Critique," *Regulation*, January-February 1981, pp. 33-40.

10. Jane S. Willems et al., "Cost Effectiveness of Vaccination against Pneumococcal Pneumonia," *The New England Journal of Medicine,* vol. 303 (1980), pp. 553-559.

11. George Akerlof "The Market for Lemons," *Quarterly Journal of Economics,* vol. 84 (1970), pp. 488-500; Michael Spence, "Job Market Signalling," *Quarterly Journal of Economics,* vol. 87 (1973), pp. 355-374.

12. See, however, Reuben A. Kessel, "Price Discrimination in Medicine," *Journal of Law and Economics,* vol. 1 (1958), pp. 20-53; Richard L. Landau, ed., *Regulation of New Drugs* (Chicago: University of Chicago Center for Public Policy, 1973), especially the paper by Sam Peltzman, "The Benefits and Costs of New Drug Regulations"; and Thomas McGuire and Burton A. Weisbrod, eds., *Economics of Mental Health* (Washington, D.C.: National Institute of Mental Health, 1981).

13. See also McGuire and Weisbrod, *Economics of Mental Health.*

14. This is virgin territory. For a recent study, however, that finds differences in behavior (though not in terms related to medical research) across ownership types in the nursing home industry, see Burton A. Weisbrod and Mark Schlesinger, "Proprietary, Nonprofit, and Governmental Organization Behavior in Markets with Asymmetric Information: An Application to Nursing Homes," Madison, Wisconsin: Institute for Research on Poverty, Discussion Paper no. 679-81, University of Wisconsin, 1982. For more general attempts to understand the role of the private nonprofit economic sector, see Weisbrod, *The Voluntary Nonprofit Sector* (Lexington, Mass.: D. C. Heath, 1977); and Henry Hansmann, "The Role of Nonprofit Enterprise," *Yale Law Journal,* vol. 89 (1980), pp. 835-901.

2

How Can We Evaluate Health Care?

Is Health Care Different?

All things are different from each other. The interesting question is not whether health care as a "commodity" is different in all respects from any other commodity but whether it is different in ways and to a degree that are relevant to the development of public policy. Can the forces of the decentralized private market be relied upon to serve "social objectives" essentially as well for health care as for most other goods and services?

To begin to answer this difficult question, we must first say something about what is meant by social objectives. Economists often have in mind only the goal of allocative efficiency. The goal of distributional equity is often overlooked or its significance minimized. Does the fact that health care can affect life itself warrant a public policy different from that generally regarded as desirable for other commodities? The answer is not obvious. Furthermore, it is complicated by two facts: (1) not all medical care is vital to life—indeed, most is not—and (2) there are other goods that, even though not necessary to the maintenance of life, are generally deemed to be sufficiently important that access to them should not be determined solely by private markets—for example, schooling and decent housing.

The term "health care" encompasses a variety of resources (physicians, nurses, drugs) provided by a variety of organizational structures (medical practitioners working on a fee-for-service basis, prepaid group practices, hospitals) and operating simultaneously in the public, private for-profit, and private nonprofit sectors. The definition of health care normally used, however, has two serious limitations.

This section is based on two previous works: (1) remarks made at a conference sponsored by the Federal Trade Commission in November 1977 (the original paper, in the form of comments on a paper by Professor Mark Pauly, was published in Warren Greenberg, ed., *Competition in the Health Care Sector* [Germantown, Md.: Aspen Systems Corporation, 1978, pp. 49-55]); and (2) a talk given in June 1981 at the Graduate Program in Hospital Administration, University of Chicago.

First, most health care analysts, although they do not define the term, are generally talking about the activities customarily associated with physicians and hospitals. Such a conception of the health care industry is too narrow a basis for determining public policy. Pharmacists, drugs, nursing homes, and halfway houses, for example, are frequently close substitutes for (and often complements of) physicians and hospitals. And the various paramedical workers, as well as the chiropractors, optometrists, and so on, also provide services that are at least partially substitutable for those of physicians. As in any industry, the boundary between what should be regarded as in and not in the health care industry is fuzzy. In my view, however, it is important that public policy recognize the breadth of resources and institutional structures that affect health and are to some degree substitutable for one another. Health care should therefore not be restricted to treatment, but should also include prevention, a use of resources that affects both the subsequent demand for treatment and the probable effectiveness of that treatment. Not only such preventive measures as vaccinations—typically administered by "medical providers"—should be considered, but also occupational and environmental factors affecting health: housing, diet, smoking, job hazards, automobile safety.

The second limitation is that the typical analysis of the health care production process is a static one, in which the state of knowledge is assumed to be fixed; the public policy questions are thus seen as how much of a given amount of knowledge should be employed, how it should be applied, and how it should be financed. Overlooked is the critical long-run issue of medical research policy. Yet even a casual glance at advances in knowledge in recent decades discloses that our health care choices today depend crucially on the resources devoted to research and development yesterday. Health care policy that disregards the link between the resources devoted to research and development and the options available for prevention and treatment will, in all likelihood, yield unfortunate and unintended results.

When economists think about whether the private market for a product functions adequately or whether social policy intervention is required to serve the public interest, an important issue is whether the consumers are well informed about the product. Consider the health care market. On the one hand, rising levels of education are making patients more skillful consumers of health care, better diagnosticians of health problems, and better able to determine whether professional help is needed. On the other hand, advances in knowledge resulting from research and development have continually expanded the ability of professionals to diagnose and treat, have provided new technology and drugs, have led to new medical and paramedical specialties, and, in general, have made the patient-consumer increasingly uncertain whether some new development has made his or her knowledge obsolete. Thus, as a result of changes in the capabilities of health care, a patient who has repeated contacts with a particular health care provider is not necessarily obtaining much useful information for evaluating the provider.

When we as economists focus on the frequency of purchase of a good, we are drawing attention to a process through which initially uninformed consumers become sufficiently expert buyers that we can conclude that a decentralized private competitive market will be an efficient supply mechanism. But if scientific knowledge is also expanding, the consumer-patient is not necessarily becoming better informed. In his or her repeat "purchases" the consumer is not obtaining a larger sample of treatment effectiveness from a given "population" of health care capability, but is sampling from a changing population—a result of scientific and engineering advances.

The issue of how well informed buyers of health care are, of course, is of fundamental importance and deserves far more study. Obviously much more is involved than the effects of research and development. To the extent that consumers are well informed, the case is strengthened for a public policy toward health care that regards it as like other "ordinary" commodities in the sense that consumers can be relied upon to buy efficiently and competition, if it is present, can be relied upon to serve the role of allocating resources efficiently.[1]

My own view is that consumers are generally rather poorly informed about the quality of health care being purchased. One major reason for my view is the difficulty consumers have in identifying the counterfactual, that is, what the situation will be if the good is not obtained. What a buyer wants to know is the difference between his state of well-being with and without the commodity being considered. For ordinary goods, the buyer has little difficulty in making such an evaluation. Not so for the bulk of health care. Because the human physiological system is an adaptive system, it is likely to correct itself and deal effectively with an ailment even without any medical services. A consumer of such services who gets better after the purchase does not know whether the improvement was because of, or even in spite of, the care that was received. If no health care services are purchased and the problem becomes worse, the consumer is generally not in a strong position to determine whether the results would have been different, and better, if certain health care had been purchased. And the consumer may learn little from experience or from friends' experience because of the difficulty of determining whether the counterfactual to a particular type of health care today is the same as it was the previous time that the consumer, or a friend, had similar symptoms. The noteworthy point is not simply that it is difficult for the consumer to judge quality before the purchase (as it also is for used cars) but that it is difficult even after the purchase.

The information issue is critical to determining whether medical care is different in a sense that justifies special public policy. A great deal of public policy in the consumer area is directed to promoting price competition and to expanding the provision of price information. But the importance of information on prices cannot be separated from the availability of information on quality. Giving consumers additional price information may not enhance efficient choice if they are poorly informed about quality. For most commodities, the assumption that consumers are well informed is sufficiently correct that government efforts to elicit information from producers and to stimulate competition on price are well founded. But for health care and certain other commodities (like legal representation and much of education) for which quality is especially difficult to judge, government policy should not be restricted to price information but should be balanced by simultaneous efforts to ensure that intelligible information on quality is widely available.

The information problem for much, but not all, of health care has given rise to a variety of mechanisms to protect the consumer. In addition to direct government regulation—for example, licensure and threats of license revocation—and a legal framework permitting malpractice suits, there are such private sector actions as professional ethics codes and nonprofit sector efforts to operate hospitals and nursing homes in the "public interest." The poorly informed patient has a demand for information, but frequently he does not know what information is needed or how valuable the information would be if he had it. As a result, he generally depends on some agent to evaluate the quality of medical care and the appropriateness of particular forms of care to his health conditions and preferences. The physician's ethics code and the nonprofit organizational form are two examples of devices ostensibly designed to ensure that the ill-informed patient can trust the provider to act in the patient's best interest. How well do such devices work? Little is known. Development of sound public policy toward medical care should recognize, however, that these mechanisms exist; they appear to differ from the devices of ordinary private profit-oriented markets, and they may well have useful roles to play in markets in which consumers must rely on experts whose judgment and advice are frequently either costly or impossible to monitor.

When the consumer information problem is recognized, the next step is to recognize that there are limits to what can be done about it—at least in the short run, until research can expand knowledge. Even medical experts are imperfectly informed about much of medical care. Allocative inefficiencies as well as inequities can develop, however, when better information is available to some persons, generally sellers, than to others, generally buyers, for this gives those with more information opportunities to take advantage of those with less, especially if the former are in positions of trust (for example, physicians and hospital administrators).

Is medical care different? Yes and no. It is different from most commodities in that (1) there is widespread interest in the distribution of access to it and (2) unlike most goods and services, it is difficult for consumers to evaluate, so that they depend heavily on experts in whom they must place their trust, frequently without ever knowing whether the trust was warranted. Nevertheless, medical care is similar to other commodities in that (1) there are other commodities the distribution of which is of general social interest and (2) there are other commodities that are difficult for consumers to evaluate even after purchase and thus require the consumer to rely on experts whose advice and actions are difficult to assess.

It is important to emphasize that medical care is not homogeneous and that some forms of it are more routine and easier to evaluate than others. I would emphasize, however, that consumers may learn little from experience in purchasing medical care, both because technological change causes actions that are optimal (or, at least, most effective) at one time not to be optimal (or most effective) later and because the ability of the human physiological system to adjust makes it very difficult for the patient-consumer to determine when an improvement (or worsening) of health is attributable to a particular medical care intervention. Thus, although price information and price competition are likely to be in the interests of consumers, a balanced public policy must deal simultaneously with quality as well as price, both by providing information to consumers and by stimulating competition. Finally, because of the consumer's difficulty in evaluating quality, careful consideration is needed of the role of such nonmarket mechanisms as ethics codes and nonprofit organizational forms and the role and effectiveness of regulatory mechanisms such as are used in the public utility field. When it is difficult for buyers to evaluate quality, the theorem of economics that more information—for example, on price—is always preferred to less need not hold.[2]

Eight Propositions Concerning the Evaluation of Health Services

What are the benefits of any program? How can those benefits be measured operationally? Is the measurement of benefits from health services different from the measurement of benefits from other programs? What are the differences between economists' and physicians' notions of the benefits from health services? The brief remarks that follow only scratch the surface of answers to these questions, which are as difficult to deal with as they are important.

1. *Evaluating health services is quite different from evaluating health.* It is well known that just as "health services" are among the variables influencing the state of health of a person, group, or society, so are diet, housing, living habits, work patterns, and so on. Not only is there a panoply of preventive measures—many of which do not involve health services (as that term is customarily defined) but do have profound effects on health—but the bulk of treatment of general illness uses self-treatment or successful nontreatment rather than health services. Thus any evaluation of the benefits or effectiveness of health services must cope with the complex problem of disentangling the effects on "health status," however defined, of those services from the effects of other variables.

2. *Determining the beneficial effects of health services requires answers to a counterfactual question:* What beneficial effects occur when some health service is used that would not have occurred without that service? One of the following must be true: (1) the health service is used, in which case we can, in principle, observe how well off (by some measures) the person is, but we cannot observe how well off he or she would have been without the service; or (2) the health service is not used, in which case we can observe (again in principle) how well off the person is without the service, but we cannot observe how well off he or she would have been with it. Statistical devices of various sorts, such as multiple regression analysis or randomized controlled experimentation, can help to estimate the difference in outcomes with and without the health service, but the resulting estimates necessarily remain probabilistic.

3. *The relation between measuring benefits and answering the counterfactual question, though not unique to health services, is far*

This is a revision of a presentation at the University of Uppsala (Sweden), Symposium on Evaluation Research and Measurement of Benefits of Health, entitled "Notes on the Evaluation of Health Services." The symposium papers were published in the *Scandinavian Journal of Social Medicine, Supplement 13: Evaluation Research and Measurement of Benefits of Health Services* (Stockholm: Almqvist & Wiksell Company, 1978).

more complicated for them than for most of the goods and services that people purchase. This is true for two principal reasons: (a) Since the human biological system cares for itself, we obviously cannot assume that it would remain static even if no health services were provided. By contrast, for example, if a flashlight functions properly after replacement of its battery with a new one, we can be confident that would not have happened without the replacement. The counterfactual for the flashlight is a situation of static equilibrium—no change. This is not the case for the health service. (b) Although a person may become ill many times during his life, the causes and circumstances will generally differ each time. This leads to the next point.

4. *The consumer of health services is a poor judge of their quality.* "Quality" is, in this context, a synonym for "benefits," whatever form they may take in the judgment of the consumer. The consumer is generally (though not always) a poorer judge than physicians of how effective a particular health service is in correcting some illness, because he does not know whether the illness would have been better or worse without the service. Patients may care, however, not only about outcomes but also about the anxiety that often accompanies illness; insofar as health services reduce anxiety, they provide a benefit quite apart from their effect, if any, on health. Reduction of anxiety is one criterion by which health services should be evaluated.

5. *Both consumers and providers of health services tend to judge benefits by the procedures used rather than by the state of health that results.* While health professionals are more expert than consumers in judging the marginal effect of a set of health services on a patient, the combination of the counterfactual problem and the self-regulating human biological system often produces considerable uncertainty, even for the experts, about the consequences of those services. Development of sound public policy needs to wrestle with the problem of how to separate health care procedures (which are easy to observe and measure but less relevant conceptually) from outcomes (which are hard to observe and measure but more relevant conceptually).

6. *The actual and potential role of professional ethics codes in the medical care market is important and not yet sufficiently understood.* The persons with the best technical knowledge for evaluating health services are the providers, because they understand better than consumers (though far from perfectly) the nature of the system in which medical care inputs operate; yet providers do not always have incentives to be self-critical or to seek out lower-cost procedures. (Providers are not always the best-informed persons; patients have

a great deal of information, but their lack of technical training limits their ability to interpret it.) Information problems are fundamental to evaluating and rationalizing the health care system. Ethics codes, at least in their more idealistic conceptions, claim to cope with possible conflicts of providers' interests in the light of (a) the consumers' difficulty in judging quality, and (b) the associated need by the consumer-patient to trust health care providers. Do the codes work at all satisfactorily and, if so, under what conditions? Or are they (as economists have tended to consider them) nothing more than monopolistic devices for reducing competition and external pressures from consumers and government?

7. *We need to learn more about how satisfactorily health care providers carry out their fiduciary role with respect to consumers.* Because of the difficulty of evaluating quality, health service providers come to act as agents for consumers—agents in whom a good deal of trust and faith are placed. Improved mechanisms are needed to give those providers the incentives to carry out their fiduciary role efficiently and equitably.

8. *Health services should not be evaluated socially against a standard of the highest quality that the state of technology permits.* Incentives such as pricing or rationing need to discourage or prevent efforts to achieve the technologically best quality of health services. The "best" is generally too costly. Technological advances now make it possible to devote enormous amounts of resources to health services, but only by incurring correspondingly enormous costs. "Costs" refer not simply to money but to the society's always limited resources. The economist's broad perspective makes it clear that higher-quality health services, though desirable, inevitably imply a lower quality or quantity of other things that consumers also want. It is not true, therefore, that any enhancement in the quality of health services is always preferred by consumers to the amounts of other goods and services that could be produced with the same resources.

It is this trade-off between health services and other uses of resources that often serves to separate the views, evaluative approaches, and policy recommendations of economists from those of physicians. Everyone recognizes the necessity to make some trade-off—the entire gross national product cannot be devoted to health services. Beyond that recognition, however, there is little agreement. This is attributable in part to difficulties in assessing the effectiveness of health services and in part to difficulties in evaluating their relative importance, even if we know their effectiveness.

Difficulties in Evaluating Health Care Markets:
The Example of Mental Health

Mental health care services are a subset of health services, but they exemplify the problems of assessing market performance in the health service area in particularly striking forms. Imagine a commodity with the following characteristics:

* The resources devoted to it are growing rapidly.

* Governments—federal, state, and local—are the principal sources of financial support for the industry that produces it.

* Private nonprofit organizations are its major providers, sometimes with their own funds but often with governmental funds.

* Its effectiveness in accomplishing what it claims to accomplish is very difficult to assess.

* New producers are entering the industry in substantial numbers, but each entrant is providing an identifiably different version of the generic commodity.

* The new producers, claiming that their products are as effective as those of the traditional producers, are struggling to have their products also covered by insurance.

* Technical change has transformed the supply side from one dominated by large government-run institutions to widely dispersed, small, more independent providers.

* The commodity is so important to some people that access to it cannot legally be denied because of the inability to pay.

* Many consumers can purchase the commodity at a price near zero because they have insurance.

* Government agencies, recognizing these conditions, are under continuous and conflicting pressure to license and not to license the new producers, to restrict entry and to facilitate competition, to expand insurance coverage to encompass some new producers and to hold down expenditures by not expanding it.

* Government agencies and private nonprofit organizations, being principal suppliers but unwilling to seek profit maximization as a goal, engage in benefit-cost analysis that is casual at best.

This is a revised version of a paper written with Thomas McGuire as an introduction to a 1979 Conference on the Economics of Mental Health, sponsored by the National Institute of Mental Health. That paper, entitled "Defining and Measuring Outputs of Mental Health Services," was published in Thomas McGuire and Burton A. Weisbrod, eds., *Economics and Mental Health*, Series EN: Mental Health Economics, No. 1, U.S. Department of Health and Human Services, National Institute of Mental Health, 1981.

Surely such a commodity, its industry, and the governmental regulatory role would attract much economic research. Treatment of mental illness is just such a commodity; yet the attention it has received from economists has been minute.

Mental illness has for some time been recognized as a serious social problem. The President's Commission on Mental Health estimated that 15 percent of the U.S. population is afflicted by mental illness during a year and called mental illness our major public health problem. The costs it imposes on victims and on society are hard to measure, but are widely acknowledged to be enormous, no doubt dwarfing the 1 percent of GNP devoted to treating it.

Why has such a serious problem received so little attention from economists? Twenty-five years ago most mental health care was provided in state and county mental hospitals, settings in which the allocation device was "professional authority"—a variable that did not seem to be amenable to analysis with the usual tools of economics. But the excuse that economists' tools do not fit the problem of resource allocation in mental health, though of some validity twenty-five years ago, is not valid today. There has been improvement in the methods of economic analysis, and, more important, there has been technical change in the mental health sector. Spurred by advances in psychopharmacology and by judicial acknowledgment of patients' rights to treatment in the "least restrictive setting," treatment for the seriously mentally ill has shifted in emphasis from long-term hospitalization to short-term hospitalization or to drug therapy and treatment in community settings without hospitalization. Over the same period larger and larger numbers of less seriously ill persons have sought to "buy" psychotherapy from an expanded range of providers.

As mental health care has moved out of the hospitals and into the community, it has increasingly shifted into settings in which markets function. The perspectives of economics, including analysis of consumers' behavior in response to price changes, analysis of suppliers' behavior in response to competition and regulation and cost-benefit analysis, can effectively be brought to bear on problems in mental health services. So far, however, this research potential is far from realized.

The lack of adequate understanding of what constitutes mental health and the lack of consensus about the effectiveness of various forms of therapy are obstacles for the economist who ventures into the mental health care area. Progress in understanding mental illness and treatment is slow; public policy is unlikely to be rescued by breakthroughs in knowledge. In the meantime, public policy must go forward to set the terms of financing and regulation of mental health services in the presence of substantial uncertainty about the ultimate benefits and costs of policy alternatives.

The lack of professional consensus about what constitutes mental health has contributed to the wariness of both private insurance companies and the government in offering coverage for mental health services. Given the combination of (1) a zero or, at least, "low" price of treatment for the patient, (2) the incentive of providers to extend treatment if they see any benefit to the patient, and (3) the patient's lack of expertise in judging the value of added therapy, the ambiguity regarding mental health provides a potential for enormous expenditures in therapy. Not surprisingly, therefore, coverage for mental illness is less than for physical illness in most private insurance plans and in most proposed national health insurance bills.

Insurers, finding it difficult to assess the effectiveness of alternative therapies but wishing to control the rate of growth of claims and rates, have faced increasing pressure to provide coverage for an ever-widening array of providers of treatment for the mentally ill. Consumers, often ill-informed about the therapeutic value of particular treatments but facing a marginal price near zero because of third-party payments, are often not constrained to use lower-cost treatments. At the same time, prospective providers with new therapeutic approaches see that there is a potential market for any innovation simply because of the relative absence of incentives for patients to economize. In many instances patients are treated by expensive covered therapies where less expensive but uncovered methods would have been at least as effective. When patients, providers, and policy makers are uncertain about the appropriate form of care, many such mismatches are likely to occur.

Difficulties in measuring output also imply difficulties in monitoring services to be sure that what is paid for is appropriate. Conventional devices to restrain overutilization, such as utilization and peer review, may work relatively badly in mental health. Experts often disagree about the appropriate course of treatment. The experts who are best informed about a particular patient are generally those who are providing the care; being involved themselves, however, they are hardly in a position to give objective counsel. Such conflicts of interest have received some attention from economists in the context of principal-agent relationships—the service provider being both an agent for his or her patient and a principal acting on his or her own behalf. The applicability of this analytic framework to mental health care seems evident.

It is just such situations, involving asymmetric information—where the service provider knows more about the quality and effectiveness of the care than the patient—that often give rise to demands for government regulation. Many regulatory mechanisms operate in the area of mental health treatment, including occupational licensure (through licensing, certification, and registration), government-mandated planning agencies for facilities, and self-policing by professional associations. How effectively each operates and under what circumstances they are more effective, or less, than such indirect regulatory mechanisms as competition in the private marketplace are challenging research questions.

Another question about which little is known that affects cost-benefit analysis in the mental health care industry is the extent to which types of mental health providers can be substitutes for one another. Mental health services have traditionally been dominated by psychiatrists. As much as any major part of the health sector, mental health has seen the dominance of physicians challenged by the rise in prestige and responsibility of other professions, notably clinical psychology, psychiatric social work, and psychiatric nursing. The substitution of these workers for psychiatrists may well be largely responsible for the dramatic fall in psychiatrists' incomes in relation to those of other physicians, although much research on such substitution remains to be done. But whether members of these professions can be substituted for psychiatrists—in the sense that they can produce the same outputs—or whether changes in personnel are simply the result of efforts to economize on expenditures by institutions the quality of whose output cannot be easily monitored is unknown.

The mode of treating the mentally ill is a critical dimension of public policy. The wisdom of the traditional dependence on long-term care has increasingly come to be questioned both by budget-conscious government officials and by mental health professionals who see institutionalization as counterproductive, as breeding dependence rather than the independence needed for daily life. Again in this context the importance—and often the perversity—of incentives becomes clear. There seems to be some tendency, for example, for hospitals and nursing homes to take advantage of the fact that governmental payments do not adequately vary with the degree of illness of the patients; providers can "cream off" the less sick patients. As economists we are familiar with the consequences of establishing a uniform price for goods or services of nonuniform quality. Some variant of Gresham's law operates, with the result that, in the case of the mentally ill, the high-cost cases receive the least attention.

Analyzing the benefits and costs of alternative therapies for mental illness poses substantial challenges both conceptually and empirically. It is difficult, as noted earlier, to specify with confidence what would happen to a particular mentally ill person if he or she had not been treated by one technique or set of inputs but had been treated by another or had not been treated at all. Determining such facts is a big enough problem, but to this must be added other difficulties, such as gaining agreement on concepts and measures of improved mental health and setting a value on effects for which either there are no market prices or the prices are deemed "inappropriate." Even when prices are available, they may not be regarded as relevant because of an ethic that willingness to pay for treatment, which reflects the person's income and wealth, should not affect access to care.

Substantial governmental and other third-party participation in the financing of mental health services has confronted patients and providers with prices that do not reflect social opportunity costs. This can cause serious distortions in benefit-cost analyses undertaken to evaluate alternative therapeutic approaches. Such analyses are essential, however, since profitability as understood in the private proprietary sector cannot be relied upon to allocate mental health resources efficiently, given the imperfect information of consumers, the absence of user charges for many services, and the quantitative importance of governmental and private nonprofit providers.

Benefit-cost analysis is difficult to apply to mental health services. It would be exactly wrong to conclude, however, that such analysis should not be vigorously pursued.[3] It is precisely for commodities such as mental health care, where consumers cannot easily weigh costs and benefits, that formal research has value. While benefit-cost analysis in the mental health area is in its infancy, the need to decide whom to treat, and how, makes unavoidable some kind of evaluation of alternatives—formal or informal, simple or elaborate. Because the technology for treating the mentally ill has undergone and is undergoing such radical change (sharp increases in the use of drugs and outpatient or community-based services and sharp decreases in long-term hospitalization), because it is difficult to define and measure benefits, and because the potential for incurring treatment costs as health insurance coverage is expanded is enormous, the importance of benefit-cost assessments of alternatives is great and growing.

All the problems I have been discussing grow out of the difficulty of gauging the effectiveness of much health and mental health care. That difficulty, together with minimal barriers to entry, has facilitated introduction of many new, sometimes exotic approaches to therapy. These new approaches have profoundly influenced the supply of various types of therapists. They have produced political pressures for occupational regulation and licensure. They have raised questions about which providers should be eligible for health care insurance. They have enhanced the practicality of community-based therapies, while posing new problems in the process. They have increased the need for benefit-cost analyses of the alternative therapeutic approaches. The policy implications and researchable questions resulting from the changing technology of mental health care are indeed striking.

Underlying all my remarks is a judgment that transactions in the mental health area are susceptible to useful analysis by economists, that consumers and producers do behave in predictable fashions, and that they can be expected to respond to incentives in systematic ways. This fundamental optimism about the tractability of decision-making processes in the mental health area should not, however, obscure the complexity of the issues: Who are the consumers of mental health care, in the sense of the decision makers—the mentally ill, their relatives, physicians, government planners, others? How well informed are consumers about the benefits and the costs of alternative therapies? To what extent do the privately perceived benefits and costs measure the social benefits and costs? How responsive are providers and consumers to changing incentives in such forms as prices, co-insurance, and deductibles? How is the behavior of the mental health care industry affected by the involvement of governments in central ways—state-run mental hospitals, community mental health clinics, federal financing of Medicare, state financing of Medicaid? How is the behavior of the industry affected by the prominence of private nonprofit organizations—in short-term hospitals and nursing homes, for example? When government providers, nonprofit organizations, and proprietary firms coexist, as they do in the nursing home and hospital industries, how does the process of adjustment to private or governmental incentives differ from what we have come to expect for an ordinary profit-maximizing industry? How has the industry been affected by court decisions that have, for example, led to the discharge of tens of thousands of persons from long-term mental hospitals?

There is indeed a fascinating variety of important issues with which public policy makers—and economists—must wrestle. Sometimes the policy issues appear in the popular media as simply budgetary. Any attempt to control expenditures, however, is likely to flounder unless it reflects understanding of the basic dimensions of economic choice discussed here: the forces affecting the demand for mental health care by patients and their agents, the forces affecting the supply of resources to the mental health care industry, the consequences of regulation of labor and capital in the industry, the problems of caring for the chronically mentally ill as they move increasingly out of hospitals and into community-based settings, and the need for benefit-cost analyses of alternative treatment approaches so as to recognize that not only expenditures but also benefits vary with governmental control measures.

One important and, in my view, underestimated force at work in shaping the health care market is the enormous expenditure over the years on medical research and development. Chapter 3 discusses in some detail the relationship between technical progress in the health area and total expenditures on health care.

Notes

1. There may still be distributional equity considerations, involving financing and access to health care, that justify public policy intervention.

2. For further elaboration of this point, though not specifically in the medical care context, see Russel Settle and Burton Weisbrod, "Governmentally Imposed Standards: Some Normative and Positive Aspects," in Ronald Ehrenberg, ed., *Research in Labor Economics*, vol. 2 (Greenwich, Conn.: JAI Press, 1978).

3. See chapter 6.

3

The Relationship between Technical Progress and Total Expenditures on Health Care

Item: The last thirty years have seen advances in medical knowledge that at the turn of this century would have been unimaginable except by science fiction writers or the most starry-eyed thinkers—organ transplants and artificial organs, vaccines that have virtually eliminated such dreaded diseases as poliomyelitis, drugs that have made possible a 75 percent reduction in the number of persons in mental hospitals since 1955 and have made massive influenza epidemics only memories.

Item: Recent years have seen explosive growth in expenditures for medical care, which have risen from 4.5 percent of gross national product (GNP) in 1950 to 7 percent in 1969 and to nearly 10 percent in 1981.

Item: During this same period there has been dramatic growth in political attention to health-care insurance.

Are these concurrent developments coincidental? We think not.

It is medical research, we suggest, that not only has brought us to a new age in our ability to prevent, detect, and successfully treat many of humankind's age-old health problems but also has played a major role in all these developments. It has slashed the mortality rates of many diseases, but often in ways that entail massive costs, which have led to a mushrooming demand for health care insurance. The insurance has reduced individual sensitivity to the rising cost of treatment and has thus brought about the increasing growth of health

A slightly different version of this paper, written with John H. Goddeeris and entitled "Medical Progress and Health Care Expenditures: The Uneasy Marriage," was published in *Viewpoints* by Hoffmann-LaRoche, Inc., 1980.

care expenditures. Medical research, then, is the source of both the advances that have dramatically reduced pain, suffering, and premature death and the escalating expenditures. Many schemes have been proposed for stemming the "inflation" of expenditures: deductibles and copayment in insurance programs, health maintenance organizations (HMOs), prospective (rather than retrospective cost-based) reimbursement schemes for hospitals, second opinions on the need for surgery, professional services review organizations (PSROs), and absolute limits on the rate of increase in expenditures are only some of the devices suggested and used. Seldom has anyone stopped to diagnose the source of the problem or to see its roots in the "successes" of medical research.

Our view, perhaps already clear, is that the fruits of medical research are mixed. The benefits of advances in medical knowledge are not without costs. Not only are there well-recognized costs of performing the research, but there are costs of applying the new knowledge. In some instances the application costs seem small, as with the one-time cost of a few dollars to administer polio vaccine to a child. In other instances the application costs seem large, as with the annual cost of $10,000 or more to provide kidney dialysis for someone with renal disease. The expenditure implications are vastly greater than these direct sums suggest, however, and the process that determines total health care expenditures is far more complex than these illustrations imply. The recipe, in short, for producing ever-growing demands on the health care budget is to add a measure of new knowledge (research) to a democratically controlled political pot. The heat will be generated either by actions to augment the supply of resources needed to use the new knowledge or by finance mechanisms (insurance) that will augment the market demand for the knowledge (since better health should not be available only to the wealthy). The addition of another measure of knowledge will keep the brew boiling.

To be clear at the outset, we are not arguing that all increases in health care expenditures brought about by medical research are undesirable or that access to costly medical treatments should be limited to those willing and able to pay. The minimization of health care expenditures should not be an overriding social objective; changes in such expenditures are a poor proxy for changes in social welfare. We do contend, however, that the full implications of medical progress, both for health care expenditures and for social welfare—that is, for total benefits as well as for social costs—have not been appreciated. A broader perspective is necessary for informed policy making.

Medical Knowledge, Insurance, and the State of Health

Why has the medical sector come to absorb an increasingly large segment of our national resources? The answer heard most often from economists has to do with the growing role of public and private insurance. Only about one-third of expenditures on medical care now comes directly out of the patient's pocket; the rest is covered by private insurance or through government programs (primarily Medicare and Medicaid). Such third-party financing leads consumers to perceive medical care as virtually costless at the time it is received and therefore to demand more expensive medical care than they would if they paid the full costs directly. At the same time, doctors and hospitals are scarcely constrained by their patients' ability to pay and are free to pursue their goals regardless of the drain on society's limited resources.

That more extensive medical insurance leads to greater expenditures on medical care is now firmly established empirically. This simple insight has contributed much to our understanding of the rise in medical expenditures over the past two decades. But we must not let it carry us away. If we take a longer view, the method of financing care cannot be considered an autonomous force that independently determines expenditures. We must ask what causes the growth in demand for medical insurance. And although one may criticize the concept of "medical need" as imprecise and difficult to quantify, it remains true that healthier people, other things equal, do tend to spend less on medical care. It follows that a population's health status—somehow defined—must be an important determinant of the quantity of resources it devotes to medical care. But also important must be the state of medical knowledge, for this affects health status as well as opportunities for using resources to prevent or treat illness. We spend far more on medical care today than we did in 1900 largely because we know more now about sickness and how to treat it. Successful research has shown us how to spend money on resources in new ways.

The three factors we have mentioned as important determinants of the level of medical expenditure—the state of medical knowledge, the methods of finance, and the health status of the population—are not independent. The persistent growth of both private insurance and public programs for financing medical expenditures in recent decades suggests that it is not a random occurrence. In 1940 less than 10 percent of the population had any health insurance; by 1950 50 percent had some coverage; now over 80 percent have private coverage, and most of the rest have governmental coverage through Medicare or Medicaid. Moreover, coverage has grown more comprehensive. Such changes in financing arrangements are to some extent a response to changes in the state of medical knowledge.

The determinants of a population's health—as measured, for example, by age-specific death rates or life expectancy—have recently received attention from epidemiologists and demographers. The results are inconclusive, although we are generally warned that medical care may be less important than diet and environment. Still, important changes in medical knowledge will, over time, affect the population's health and consequently its need and economic demand for medical care.

We are arguing, then, that the state of medical knowledge is a fundamental determinant of the level of medical expenditure and that over time it influences expenditures through various channels. Stated somewhat differently, the total medical care expenditures in a particular year are determined by the interaction of financing arrangements, the medical needs of the population, and the state of medical knowledge. All these factors are changing; we focus attention here on the state of knowledge, because it influences the other two.

What influences the state of knowledge? This is another complex question, but it is clear that we as a nation exert influence on the rate and direction of growth of knowledge by our decisions on the allocation of resources to medical research. Since decisions about medical research may be influenced by financing arrangements for medical care and by the medical needs of the population, the system in which medical expenditures are determined can be regarded as a simultaneous one involving medical research, insurance, and the state of health of the population.

From the Growth of Medical Knowledge to the Demand for Insurance. Medical research has come a long way in a relatively short time. The overview cluster of the President's Biomedical Research Panel summarized the progress of medicine:

> Fifty years ago the term technology, and for that matter science, would have seemed incongruous in a discussion of medical practice. The highly skilled practitioner was a master of diagnostic medicine, but the ultimate intentions of his skill were limited to the identification of the particular illness, the prediction of the likely outcome, and then the guidance of the patient and his family while the illness ran its full, natural course. . . .
> During the past quarter-century, the life sciences have

extended into areas of human knowledge not known to exist before that time. Entirely new disciplines have emerged almost overnight, a research technology has evolved with the sophistication and power to match, almost, that achieved earlier by the physical sciences, and because of all this, the profession of medicine has begun to experience a transformation unlike anything in the millennia of its existence.[1]

It is more than mere chance that, as the power of medicine has grown, so also has the role of private and public insurance. Advances in treatment methods have created a situation in which very large expenditures appear to make a difference—sometimes a life-and-death difference—in treating some illnesses. Therefore to a greater extent than ever in the past, individuals would not be able to pay for treatments perceived as valuable unless they were aided by some form of insurance. Growth of knowledge has thus created demand for insurance.

The growth of private medical insurance should be seen partly as a response to the expansion of knowledge. Individuals found that they could guarantee themselves access to very expensive procedures if they pooled their risk with others. For the elderly and the poor, groups that have difficulty paying the premiums necessary to ensure them access to care comparable to that received by the rest of society, public programs were developed.

The direct benefits of the principal public programs, Medicare and Medicaid, accrue to a minority of the population (albeit a large one), while the costs are borne by taxpayers in general. A cynical explanation for the existence of such programs is that they (like protective tariffs) provide sizable benefits to well-defined groups having substantial political power while the costs are diffused across the population. The beneficiaries therefore lobby for them strongly, and the rest of us do not care enough to put up opposition. But in the case of medical care that explanation is far from the whole story. Support for the concept of helping the poor and aged pay for medical care runs far beyond those directly benefiting. As a society we may accept inequality of incomes generally, but we are less comfortable in allowing some people to die or to suffer pain simply because they cannot afford the medical care available to others. In a democratic society, significant medical advances create pressure for financing arrangements that will make the innovations available to all who need them. Thus the timing of the introduction of Medicare and Medicaid, in our view, had much to do with the great progress in medicine that had begun only a couple of decades earlier.

From New Knowledge to Medical Expenditures. We often think of technological change—the application of advances in knowledge—as reducing the cost of producing goods and services. Yet advances in medicine often increase expenditures on the illnesses to which they apply. This is no paradox, for in such cases the nature of the product itself changes. Higher expenditures are accepted, presumably, because they are perceived as a price worth paying for better treatment. But medical advances do not always increase expenditures. Sometimes they are both more effective and less costly than the measures they replace, as was polio vaccine, which substituted, to some extent, for the iron lung.[2] Or they may be so much less costly as to be accepted even though they appear to be slightly less effective.

Lewis Thomas, in *The Lives of a Cell*, classifies the state of medical knowledge with respect to treatment of illnesses into three categories.[3] The first category he calls "nontechnology." This refers to the supportive, nonspecific kind of care that is given when little is known about how to deal effectively with some condition. As the quotation from the President's Biomedical Research Panel indicates, medicine was in general at the nontechnology stage early in this century. We are still at this stage with respect to some diseases, notably stroke, cirrhosis, and some forms of cancer.

Thomas labels the second category "halfway technology." By that he means measures taken "to compensate for the incapacitating effects of certain diseases whose course one is unable to do much about." Halfway technologies are directed at the symptoms of illnesses whose underlying mechanisms are not yet well understood. Many of the best-known advances of the last twenty years have been of a halfway nature. Machines that take over the function of some failed bodily organ provide one striking kind of example. Most therapies currently available for treating cancer and heart disease are halfway measures. Surgical removal of cancerous tissues, for example, is a desperate measure performed because we do not know how to prevent or reverse the disease process.

The final category is the truly decisive "high technology," which "comes as a result of a genuine understanding of disease mechanisms." Such technology usually takes the form—at least in the examples Thomas gives—of a vaccine or drug. Among his examples are the modern treatments of tuberculosis and typhoid fever and the prevention of poliomyelitis and diphtheria.

Movements from the nontechnology to the halfway technology stage are frequently associated with increased expenditures. The iron lung for polio victims and the kidney dialysis machinery for victims of renal diseases produced enormous increases in medical expendi-

FIGURE 3–1

HEALTH EXPENDITURES AND THE STATE OF TECHNOLOGY

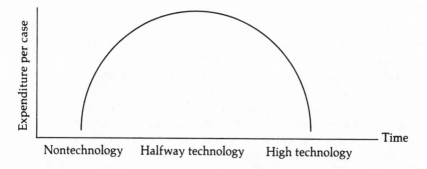

tures, since before their development knowledge was so limited that there was virtually no way to devote substantial resources to treatment.

When high technologies are developed, Thomas argues, they are not only more effective but invariably less costly than the treatments they replace. This seems very probable if the high technology replaces a halfway technology, although the evidence we have so far is little more than anecdotal. But if high technology replaced a nontechnology state of knowledge, it is by no means self-evident that medical expenditures would be reduced.

Thomas's three states of technology, or knowledge, suggest to us a hypothesis regarding the long-run evolution of knowledge. Viewed from a perspective of many decades or even centuries, the development of medical knowledge about how to prevent or treat any disease and the average expenditure required to prevent or treat it may be hill-shaped (see figure 3–1).

Such a pattern characterized the historical development of knowledge about poliomyelitis. At the nontechnology stage, expenditures were probably low: many victims died immediately, and there was little potential for spending funds to treat the permanently crippled. But expenditures grew as a halfway technology, the iron lung, was developed. Now the development of low-cost, effective vaccines has cut expenditures on polio sharply.

At any time, the state of knowledge places some illnesses at relatively low-expenditure points on their respective "hills" (whether at the nontechnology or the high-technology stage) and other illnesses at high expenditure points. Total health care expenditures depend, therefore, on the particular constellation of knowledge stages existing at the time. Does our recent experience with rapidly rising expenditures on medical care reflect medical research taking us from the nontechnology or "low" technology stage to a halfway technology more often than from halfway to high technology? If so, we may yet look forward to an era of diminishing medical care expenditures as knowledge moves us increasingly to the high-technology stage.

In short, the recent enormous increases in medical expenditures may be more a temporary bulge than the beginnings of a trend likely to continue indefinitely. It seems reasonably clear that innovations in medical practice in the last several decades have been largely of the halfway variety and have contributed significantly to rising expenditures. Perhaps the halfway measures are only a temporary stopping place before advances in the understanding of disease produce low-cost cures or preventive measures for far more illnesses.

Such optimism must be tempered by several considerations. First, even if medical research soon yields the high technologies that will control major illnesses, we have little assurance that they will be inexpensive to apply. If an illness becomes preventable through immunization, for example, the cost per case prevented may be quite high if the illness itself is rare. If the entire adult population, over 200 million persons, must be vaccinated for a disease that would otherwise have struck only one in 10,000, the relevant comparison is between the cost of 200 million vaccinations and the cost of treating 20,000 cases.

Second, and more fundamental, the effect of a given technological change on medical expenditures depends on the time perspective we take. Most discussions of the effects of a technological change on expenditures confine attention to the effect on the treatment costs of the particular illness involved. But a change in treatment method—by changing the outcome of the illness—will generally influence the patient's lifetime pattern and level of medical expenses.

To see how changes in lifetime expenditures on health care can vary quite independently of the changes in direct expenditures, consider the example of an innovation in treatment that cures a previously fatal illness. Imagine a world, for example, with a constant birthrate in which individuals live for at most two periods. Ninety percent are healthy in the first period; the other 10 percent contract pneumonia and die. All those who survive into the second period eventually die of cancer. Treatment of pneumonia costs ten dollars, of cancer one hundred dollars. Now suppose that research produces a new treatment that cures pneumonia at a cost of only one dollar. The immediate effect of the innovation is to reduce medical expenditures. But in the second period after the innovation is adopted, medical expenditures are higher both in total and on average over the lifetime of an individual.

38

The example is simple, but the idea is important. Given that death remains inevitable, any research that succeeds in preventing or controlling one kind of fatal illness necessarily increases the probability that we will eventually contract others. The great success of medical science in controlling infectious illnesses such as tuberculosis, pneumonia, and diphtheria has meant that people now die—more slowly and expensively—from illnesses like cancer and heart disease.

The point is that the full effect of new knowledge on an individual's lifetime medical expenditures can be, and generally is, vastly different from the immediate effects. The difference may be in either direction. A person may be saved from one disease at low cost only to die later after incurring far greater costs. By contrast, a person who is prevented from contracting some disease or is cured of it may be less likely to contract some other disease that is more costly to treat. Prevention of scarlet fever among children, for example, leaves persons who would have been its victims but would not have died from it stronger and less susceptible to complications associated with a weakened heart, complications for which a costly treatment technology exists. Thus, although a lifetime perspective reminds us that every person will die, total lifetime medical care expenditures may be increased or decreased by medical advances. We want to emphasize that the lifetime expenditure effect of medical research need not be positively correlated with its effect on expenditures for the illness that it prevents or treats.

From Methods of Financing Care to the Growth of Knowledge. Thomas's references to halfway technologies and our discussion of stages in technological evolution suggest that these are intermediate steps that must be taken before the final high technology can be reached. But the development of radiation therapy and sophisticated surgical procedures—both halfway technologies—for cancer treatment have contributed little to our understanding of the underlying causes of the disease; they do not seem to have brought us closer to an inexpensive high technology. Nor has the development of coronary bypass surgery brought us any closer to effective prevention of arteriosclerosis. One may ask, then, why we have seen the development of so many halfway technologies and so few high technologies. Why do we not more often skip the intermediate step entirely and move directly to the high-technology stage?

To some it may seem absurd even to raise such questions. They would argue that scientific progress simply proceeds as it does and we can neither predict nor control it. We do not accept that view. Society devotes substantial funds to medical research—more than $3 billion per year, of which more than $2.5 billion is from the National Institutes of Health (NIH) alone—and it makes careful and deliberate decisions on how to allocate them. These actions imply a belief that by our decisions about which research to support we can influence the speed and direction of scientific progress.

No one would deny that, given the underlying base of scientific knowledge available at any time, some lines of research are more promising than others. Nonetheless, which problems get solved—which innovations are developed—is influenced not only by the difficulty of the problems but also by the amounts of effort devoted to their solution. In research as elsewhere, we face the economic problem of allocating scarce resources to competing ends. Should we devote most of our efforts to applied problems that appear solvable in the short run, or should we concentrate heavily on more difficult problems whose solutions would ultimately be of greater value? What portion of our efforts ought to be devoted to more basic scientific research, aimed at altering over a longer period of time the knowledge base on which applied research must build? These questions are alternative ways of asking what quantity of resources should go into developing halfway technologies that, once developed, will impose large and politically irresistible demands on the public budget—witness the development of kidney dialysis technology with current annual expenditures of more than $1 billion for making it available to all who can benefit from it—and what quantity should go into research that reaches out for low-cost solutions to health problems.

Innovation in the private sector normally responds to the demand for it. The greater the value of any innovation to users—and therefore the greater the potential profit for the developers—the more likely that the research necessary for development will be undertaken. Whether a profit motive is as relevant to medical research as to other areas of production is less obvious. Although there is a sizable investment in medical research by profit-making firms (largely pharmaceutical companies), about two-thirds of medical research is financed by government, and another significant segment is funded by nonprofit organizations. Such research is performed mainly by scientists working for government or for universities that are not profit oriented.

Nonetheless, government, in selecting what research projects to finance, and scientists, in choosing what lines of research to pursue, are influenced not only by perceptions of the likelihood of success in various areas but also by beliefs about the potential value of different types of medical advances. Thus demand affects the allocation of effort to research even in health care and ultimately affects the direction of technological change in medicine.

40

We can now see how the existing financing arrangements for medical care influence the pattern of research and the innovations that emerge. The presence of health insurance and other financial arrangements under which consumers can afford extremely expensive medical procedures makes research aimed at developing them more attractive to researchers as well as to firms. The growth of insurance and other collective financing arrangements has deflected the path of research and innovation in a direction that increases expenditures on treatment. In the process the development of costly halfway technologies has been made more attractive to scientists and more profitable to private firms than they would have been in the absence of the various third-party payment arrangements. Knowledge about health and disease is always limited. How such knowledge will be used depends on the incentives that exist. Expansion of insurance-type payment mechanisms has strengthened incentives to apply knowledge to expenditure-increasing rather than to expenditure-reducing technological change. This is an unforeseen result of efforts to make the benefits from medical advances more widely accessible.

Conclusion

Society's goals often conflict. Our society has not adequately recognized the degree to which encouraging medical innovation, making the fruits of the new knowledge available to all regardless of ability to pay, and holding down the costs of medical care are incompatible. It is only somewhat of an exaggeration to say that the explosion of medical care expenditures is caused by the successes of medical research. They have made possible miraculous new cures, preventives, and treatments, but often at enormous cost. Political dynamics set in motion by these new opportunities have succeeded in making them widely accessible even though their cost-effectiveness is often unclear; witness the current controversy over the effectiveness of coronary bypass surgery in reducing heart attacks. At the same time that the new financing mechanisms are succeeding in their goal of broadening access to the "best" medical care, they are not only generating rapid rises in medical care expenditures but also shifting incentives for subsequent research. No longer need researchers be concerned about whether their discoveries will find a market. High costs and the resulting high prices generally deter widespread adoption of innovations in the economy. To the extent, however, that high-cost technologies need not meet a private market test of willingness and ability to pay because a political test has been met, more resources will flow toward research leading to such technologies. Passing a political rather than a private market test is not necessarily undesirable; it is different, however, and it gives researchers incentives to seek higher-cost innovations.

Conflicting goals imply a dilemma. A crucial element in coping with the dilemma of health care expenditures and medical innovations is recognition of the centrality of medical research. Its nature and direction are simultaneously a cause of rising medical care expenditures and a result of the mechanisms used to finance those expenditures.

Notes

1. President's Biomedical Research Panel, Report, App. A, 1976.
2. See chapter 5.
3. New York: Bantam Books, 1975.

4

Benefit-Cost Analysis in the Health Area: Issues and Directions for Research

Introduction

Development of sound public policy in any program area requires two types of knowledge: an understanding of what consequences will follow from a particular course of action, and an evaluation of the desirability of those consequences. The first involves "positive" analysis—*description* of how the relevant economic, social, political, biological, or other system functions. The second involves "normative analysis" —*assessment* of how favorable or unfavorable the effects of some intervention will be.

Benefit-cost analysis is a framework for the latter, normative analysis. It is useful for assessing the advantages and disadvantages of decisions made outside the private sector, outside the realm of which private profitability is an acceptable indicator of social desirability. The objectives of this paper are to identify important difficulties in applying the benefit-cost framework to evaluation of health programs—especially mental health—and, by so doing, to improve future program evaluations and to identify issues for research.[1]

The Benefit-Cost Evaluation Framework

Proposals and, indeed, actual programs abound to prevent illness, to cure those who can be cured, and to care for those who cannot be treated. In every case it would be useful to know more about the desirable and undesirable characteristics of any health care program— that is, about its benefits and costs.

This is a revision of a paper, written with Mark Schlesinger, and appearing in Thomas McGuire and Burton Weisbrod, eds., *Economics and Mental Health*, Series EN: Mental Health Economics, no. 1, U.S. Department of Health and Human Services, National Institute of Mental Health, 1981.

At an abstract level, the benefit-cost analytic problem is to discover whether the discounted present value of benefits from some programs exceeds the discounted present value of its costs. This is not controversial. Difficulties surface rapidly, however, as one begins to specify: (a) what precise forms benefits and costs take, (b) how (or whether) to place monetary values on them, what time pattern they will take, and at what interest rate to discount future benefits and costs. Since the health area poses no unusual issues in this latter regard, this chapter will not deal with the issue of what discount rate should be used, although the choice of a rate can have a profound effect on the calculation of a program's net present value.[2]

We will look at the problems and pitfalls on the benefit side of the ledger. First, however, there are some broad issues that encompass both the cost and benefit sides.

General Issues

The Counterfactual. Whatever the goals may be for some social program, the benefit-cost analyst must attempt to determine whether the achievement of those goals would be affected by the particular program. That is, the analyst must compare what will happen if the program is undertaken with the counterfactual—what would happen if the program were not undertaken. It is often wrong to assume that certain things the program would do would not otherwise be done in the absence of the program. To illustrate: A program that involves treating mentally ill people in a residential institutional setting—for example, a mental hospital—will involve "costs" of providing food. The persons involved would eat, however, even if the hospitalization were terminated. Thus, insofar as both the hospital program and its alternative (that is, its counterfactual) involve the same food cost, there is no program effect on that particular cost variable. This principle of including in costs or benefits only those consequences that would not occur in the absence of the program is of fundamental importance in program evaluation. It underscores the need for an explicit statement of the alternative with which the program being evaluated is being compared.

For the food cost example given above, the issue is transparent and the correction easily made. The principle is no less sound for the evaluation of benefits, but it may be more difficult to apply. Assume that we are valuing a program against the counterfactual of no program, and that over time participants in the program show a clear improvement (however measured) in mental health. Even though the counterfactual is no organized program, we cannot value the benefits of a program relative to the patients' initial mental health status; that is, the relevant comparison is "with" versus "without" a particular intervention, not before versus after that intervention. Even if the individuals had not participated in the particular program they might still have improved over time, either through natural means, or by seeking out aid from other sources.[3]

Controlled experiments. One valuable research approach that deals clearly with the specification of the counterfactual is the randomized control experimental design. When some patients are assigned to one treatment program, for example, and some to another, it is clear which counterfactual is being assumed; each program is being compared with the other. The randomized experimental design approach to identifying consequences of a program is not without its critics,[4] but the point to be underscored here is that this experimental design deals unambiguously with the specification of a counterfactual comparison alternative.

Controlled experiments are not always efficient. They take time and use resources; thus their costs may or may not be exceeded by their benefits. Even when controlled experiments are efficient, however, they are not always—or even often—likely to be available to a researcher-evaluator. When a treatment has come to be widely accepted as effective even though no randomized clinical experiment has been performed—for example, the "Pap" smear test for cervical cancer—a liberal society cannot, for political reasons, conduct randomized trials by withholding "effective" therapy.[5]

Natural experiments. When controlled trials are not possible, or are too costly, benefits and costs may be studied in "similar" populations in which some members have received particular treatment and others have not. Difficulties with such studies rest largely on the problems associated with selection bias. If the persons using a particular therapy have selected themselves for the treatment, or have been selected for it by experts (say, physicians) who deem it to be the best treatment for them, a comparison of them with persons who did not use the therapy tends to produce upward-biased estimates of net benefits from it.

How the success of a therapy can make it impossible to examine its effectiveness in a natural experimental setting is illustrated by a benefit-cost evaluation of an anti-ulcer drug (described in chapter 7). The drug, Tagament, was subjected to randomized clinical trials as part of the process of gaining FDA approval. That approval, however, was based on criteria of "safety" and "efficacy"—not on a benefit-cost comparison of the drug with other anti-ulcer therapies. The counterfactual that is implicit in the FDA approval process is that the affected person would receive no treatment at all. The potential for comparing the benefits and costs of Tagament with those of any other therapy is quickly disappearing. The drug is proving so successful that its penetration rate—the proportion of cases of duodenal ulcers in which it is being prescribed—is approaching 100 percent. Even though it will never reach 100 percent, evaluation of its benefits and costs will increasingly run into problems of selectivity bias as ulcer patients who do not use the drug become increasingly rare and therefore increasingly likely to be systematically different from those who do. Comparisons between users and nonusers (or users of other therapies such as surgery) will thus become less and less satisfactory as an approximation of a randomized assignment of ulcer patients among alternative therapies.

A second problem with natural experiments is that often more variables change than the experimenter-analyst can deal with systematically. For instance, a number of analyses comparing the effectiveness of a treatment regime used at one time to one prevailing at another ignored changes in other aspects of care: for instance, the increased use of antipsychotic drugs between the earlier and later periods.[6] In short, in a natural experiment it is often difficult if not impossible to control for all relevant variables other than those being studied; as a result it is easy to mistake effects of the new therapy for effects of other variables that also influence mental health and that are correlated with usage of the new therapy. (This is the econometric "omitted variable" problem.)

My general point is that random assignment is not the only experimental design likely to bear fruit in economic evaluation work in the health area. Natural experiments can also be useful, although they, too, pose problems. An evaluator can compare benefits and costs for persons using different therapies—at different times or at the same time—if careful examination of the patients' characteristics, especially those involving severity of the disease and other variables affecting the degree of success of any treatment variable, discloses no substantial differences among the patient groups.

Multiple therapies. In the preceding paragraph I implied that there might be a multiplicity of therapies available. Thus, a number of different counterfactuals need to be examined if a complete benefit-cost evaluation is to be done. Not that a single researcher can compare the benefits and costs of each actual or proposed health program with all other actual or proposed alternatives—but recognition of the multiple alternatives reminds us of the overall dimensions of the benefit-cost evaluation task.

46

A recent benefit-cost evaluation of a randomized experiment in treating the mentally ill (the "Mendota Experiment"—chapter 6) illustrates the problems and challenges associated with recognition of multiple alternatives. The program being evaluated focused on treatment in the community rather than in a traditional hospital setting.[7] The experimental treatment approach involved bringing a wide variety of psychiatric and other helping services to the patient, who lived in a normal community environment. An elaborate, multidimensional benefit-cost comparison of the two treatment approaches was undertaken. However high the quality of the benefit-cost analysis, the fact remains that the hospital-based treatment was compared with only one counterfactual, the particular set of services that characterized the experimental program. Because that program involved changing many variables simultaneously, we could not learn how the program's benefits and costs would appear if they were examined against some other therapeutic approach. To what extent were the greater benefits attributable to living conditions, to greater efforts to find jobs for the patients and to keep them at work, to providing support services at times of emotional stress, to assistance in establishing social contacts, and to the interactions among these variables as well as other treatment variables that differed between the experimental and control programs? Answering such questions is beyond the scope of any single study, but noting its relevance for policy analysis serves to heighten awareness of the nonroutine character of the benefit-cost analyst's task.

Disaggregating programs. The counterfactual to one treatment program is not necessarily the same for the whole treatment group; it may be different treatments for various "types" of patients. As between two alternative treatment modes, one may be more beneficial and/or less costly than the other for older patients, for males, for persons with particular backgrounds, and so on. In the Mendota mental health experiment, for example, large systematic differences were found between the benefits (and the costs) of the two treatment modes, depending on the patients' illness diagnoses—schizophrenics, other psychotics, and persons with personality disorders. Patients are themselves inputs to the treatment process; it is not surprising, therefore, that applying the same resources to treating patients with varying diagnoses will produce varying benefits. Research that recognizes such diversity as part of the benefit-cost evaluation is greatly needed.

Time patterns of benefits and costs. It was pointed out above that one dimension of a benefit-cost analysis is that of time. A mental health treatment program, for example, is likely to involve costs of

47

resources that continue over an extended period of time, and benefits that are lagged and of uncertain duration. Certain complications result for benefit-cost analyses, and they call for care in research: (1) Whether a controlled or natural experimental design is employed, the problem remains of predicting flows of benefits and costs beyond the period of observation. For example, it certainly cannot be assumed, without further study, that observed benefits would continue undiminished into the future if treatment were terminated or, for that matter, even if costs were incurred at a constant real level. (2) Even if the flows of benefits and costs over the "lifetime" of a project were known, it would be important for benefit-cost analysis to develop generalizations about the time patterns of the benefits and costs of "typical" programs of that type. Since the discounting process reflects a social preference for obtaining benefits sooner and for deferring costs, research that identifies conditions under which a program's benefits will be realized sooner and its costs incurred later would be useful.

Identifying the counterfactual—a conceptual note. Any benefit-cost analysis is a comparison of two states of the world. Since at most one of those states can actually exist, it follows that the other must be hypothetical. To be relevant for informing policy making, however, the hypothetical state that is assumed must be realistic, and this may pose subtle but critical problems. An illustration is instructive.

Consider a program that is 100 percent effective in curing persons with some type of mental illness. Assume that the analyst knows everything worth knowing about the current conditions of the person with that illness. What should be assumed, however, about the counterfactual situation if the treatment program is used? Specifically, is the assumption made that persons who are "cured" will be the same, in all relevant dimensions, as they would have been if they never had been ill? Such an assumption, while plausible, is quite likely to be wrong, even if the cure left absolutely no effects of the illness from a medical point of view. Attitudes of the former patient may have been affected by the illness and cure; and attitudes of others toward the former patient may also have been affected by, for example, the "stigmatizing" effect of having been mentally ill. Such attitudinal effects can cause the counterfactual of a successfully treated person to differ significantly from that of an otherwise identical person who had never been ill.[8]

The general point is that the "well-being" of a person is a function of variables reflecting (a) objective circumstances such as health

48

state and productive potential, and (b) subjective attitudes that can affect the person's access to jobs, friends, and outsiders. A successful medical treatment program may affect group (a) variables without affecting group (b) variables, or vice versa.

Real Benefits and Costs versus Money Flows: Efficiency and Equity Considerations. Perhaps the easiest error to make in benefit-cost analyses is to identify benefits or costs with exchanges of money. There can be exchanges of money and yet no benefits or costs from a social point of view. And there can be social benefits or costs without any flow of money.

That transfer of money is neither a necessary nor a sufficient condition for identifying or measuring social benefits and costs has important implications, some of which take on special importance in the health care area even though they are not unique to that area: "Economic transfer payments" should be distinguished from real social benefits and costs, and should be excluded from the efficiency component of the benefit-cost analysis. Reflecting redistributions of income, transfers are relevant to a benefit-cost program evaluation only to the extent that the goals of the program include income redistributions. Many public programs in the health field do appear to have goals that include redistribution of resources in favor of low-income persons. The well-to-do may be assumed to be able to realize the need for health services, and to have the financial ability to obtain it; the poor, however, are often believed to be poorly informed and financially "unable" to obtain certain "basic" services involving health, and a social judgment has been made to increase their access to those services.

These observations suggest a number of major researchable questions:

• How well-informed are people about how they can benefit from various health services?
• How well-informed are they about prices and availability of these services?
• Does availability of information regarding usefulness, price, and availability differ systematically across income levels and social class?
• Is there "widespread" support for including some health services in a set of "basic social needs" that should be available and financially accessible to all?[9] If so, which health services, and in what quantities?
• To what extent are publicly provided or publicly financed health services used unequally by persons with different family, occupational, and socioeconomic class backgrounds?

49

• Do benefits from given health services vary systematically with income and social class?

The general thrust of these research questions is toward building income distributional effects into benefit-cost evaluation of public programs in health. Noneconomists often criticize benefit-cost analysis for omitting the distributional dimension to benefit-cost evaluation, and in my judgment it is a valid criticism, especially in the area of health and social welfare. Even in the areas of highway construction and water resources, however, distributional consequences are generally relevant to overall project assessment, regardless of the stated "goals" of the program.[10]

Comprehensiveness of Benefit-Cost Framework. Consider a prospective health program that would bring costs and benefits in rather different forms from those of the counterfactual program. If the benefit-cost framework is not broad enough to encompass all of these forms, one program may be estimated to be more beneficial or less costly than the other even though the benefits and costs have merely changed forms, not overall magnitudes.

An illustration: an alleged cost of locating halfway houses for the mentally ill in residential communities (the type of facility currently being subsidized through a new HUD/HEW program), compared with keeping the patients in a hospital or in some other (counterfactual) location insulated from the community, is that the "normal" residents may be inconvenienced, made uncomfortable, or, conceivably, physically abused. Unless a broad, comprehensive perspective is taken, the benefit-cost analyst might count the reduced cost of hospitalization as a benefit (or, what is precisely equivalent, a cost reduction) resulting from the program, but might fail to count the burdens on other people as costs (negative benefits). Such errors would lead to biased results. The nature, direction, and magnitude of the bias would likely depend on whether the benefits or costs accrue in money form, because the nonmonetary program consequences are more easily overlooked.

Even if the consequences are in money form, however, the likelihood of overlooking some form of benefit or cost is not small. If the effect is indirect or is external to the perspective of the principal resource suppliers, it may be unnoticed. Thus, a study of the costs and benefits of treating the mentally ill in the "community" might overlook the fact that such treatment may involve some hospitalization for acute episodes of mental illness; if the benefit-cost analyst does not obtain data on hospital utilization among mentally ill patients who normally live in the community, but does obtain such data for patients whose basic mode of treatment is in the hospital, an obvious bias results.

Whenever a specific example of a potential error is given, as was done above, the danger to be avoided is clear. Nevertheless, this problem is very real, and it is relatively simple to find analyses of health care which omit such important cost factors as: (1) the cost of nonprogram treatments; (2) the costs of time to the participant; and (3) the burdens imposed on the family of the participant.[11] Thus, an accounting system must identify as comprehensively as possible a list of potential forms of benefits or costs from the project under consideration, and then seek quantitative measures of their magnitudes. Having such a list minimizes the probability that a difference in the forms of costs or benefits as between two programs will be mistakenly seen as a difference in total magnitudes.

Development of a comprehensive accounting framework will also minimize the likelihood of confusing a real benefit or cost with a pecuniary, distributional effect. With a narrower framework an analyst may discover that some persons are made worse off—that is, some private cost is incurred—but a more comprehensive accounting might disclose that such a cost is precisely offset (at least in money terms) by a benefit to other persons.

Measurability. Much of the criticism of benefit-cost analysis centers on charges that economists often measure what they can, and then disregard those conceptually relevant variables that they are unable to measure. Insofar as our injunction to be comprehensive in identifying forms of benefits and costs is followed, the analyst will find it more difficult to disregard any forms of benefits or costs simply because of measurement problems. That is desirable; it is, in fact, the principal reason for desiring such a framework.

Measurement should be distinguished from valuation. Ideally, all forms of benefits and costs would be measured in some common unit for comparison. Money is such a unit, but its importance is no greater than that of any other standard unit. While measurement of all benefits and costs in a commeasurable unit is desirable for determining whether the total benefits or total costs are greater, that measurement will not be attainable in most real program analyses. Under typical circumstances, some forms of benefits and costs that have been identified as relevant to a comprehensive framework will not permit valuation in money units (at least not in a way deemed to be satisfactory by an economist); some, however, will be measurable in quantitative though nonmoney terms. Others will not be measurable in any quantitative units.

All three of these situations were illustrated in the Mendota study, where some variables were measured in value terms (hospital treatment costs), some in quantitative but not value terms (number of arrests, number of deaths), and some, not measured at all, were highlighted by a question mark in the benefit-cost analysis summary table (for example, burdens on neighbors and coworkers). The analyst can be "proud" of the question marks; they point up the inevitable incompleteness of the analysis, and they direct attention to the specific variables that have been identified as important without being assigned an objective value.

In short, structuring the benefit-cost analysis is one step; employing the structure to measure and value the variables once identified, is another. An important example of a variable that is easy to identify, more difficult to measure, and still more difficult to value is the number of lives saved or lost by some program. While values of human life might be presented utilizing one or another valuation procedure,[12] an alternative would be simply to state the expected number of lives involved (and also, perhaps, the variance), thereby leaving it to some decision maker to provide, explicitly or implicitly, the value weight that will permit comparison with other variables.

To say there is no satisfactory measure in pecuniary terms is not to say that any variable is, in principle, immeasurable. For some variables, however, either the conceptual foundation for measurement may be too weak to justify our presenting a pecuniary measure or the costs of implementing the measure may be too high. For the same reasons, some variables will not be measured even in quantitative nonpecuniary terms; a qualitative (algebraic sign) indicator will sometimes be the optimal measure, for example, for the burdens on community members when the mentally ill live in residential areas. Finally, as noted earlier, for some variables there will be no explicit measurement at all; for these, a question mark in a tabulation of benefits and costs is the best that can be done.

The inevitable measurement fact is that the available data will rarely, if ever, meet precisely the benefit-cost analyst's requirements. Thus, it follows that:

• Although it is marginal benefits and costs that are relevant conceptually in any benefit-cost analysis, the most readily available data will almost certainly be averages.

• Averages derived from accounting records are often biased estimates of true social averages.

The use of averages derived from accounting records is "justified" largely by their relatively low-cost availability, but easy availability is only one relevant consideration for choosing data. Study is needed of the likely direction and magnitude of biases that result from the use of unadjusted accounting data, as well as the prospects for obtaining improved data.

The limitations of accounting data for benefit-cost analyses can be of major consequence. Publicly owned land and buildings, for example, are often used for health care programs. In accounting practice the opportunity cost of public land is normally disregarded and depreciation of public buildings is artificially low because it is based on historic cost. In the Mendota experiment, for example, adjustment of the state of Wisconsin's cost accounting data for the State Mental Hospital to account for publicly owned land and the depreciation costs of public buildings led to an increase of some 40 percent. Another often-overlooked class of resources involves donations of goods and services, especially volunteer labor. These may be costless to the program, but they are certainly not costless to society. According to the 1976 *Survey of Institutionalized Persons*, the ratio of volunteer to full-time paid employees is 3:4 for psychiatric hospitals, for example, and 6:5 for institutions for the mentally handicapped. Research would be useful on the role and valuation (in opportunity cost terms) of volunteer labor in health programs, and the substitutability and complementarity of such labor for other resource inputs.

Limitations of Benefit-Cost Analysis. Whatever the precise character of the proposed program, resources for its benefit-cost analysis will be limited and will constrain the analysis. In the Mendota experiment, for example, budget constraints limited the scope of the experiment in two ways: (1) in the duration of the experiment, and (2) in the opportunity to vary and control different combinations of resource inputs. In any realistic (nonexperimental) application of the community-based program, patients would not likely be restricted to fourteen months of participation as they were in the experiment (the E program); thus the experimental design permitted only conjecture regarding whether the E program's success or its costs per patient year would be different for a program of different duration.

The E treatment approach involved not one but many simultaneous differences from the traditional (the C approach) one: (a) patients were not hospitalized; (b) they lived and worked in the community; (c) people with whom patients were likely to come in contact were asked not to treat them differently from others because they were mental patients; (d) efforts were made by the E-group staff to help patients find and retain jobs; (e) E-group staff helped patients to budget their money; (f) E-group staff accompanied patients to social activities; and (g) E-group staff assisted patients in a variety of other ways that were not available to C-group patients.

Because so many treatment variables were being altered simultaneously—as is likely in all studies—any comparison of costs or benefits of the E and C programs could show only the overall net effect of altering the entire set of variables. As a theoretical ideal (abstracting from the costs of running multiple experiments), it would be desirable to run a set of experiments in which one treatment variable at a time was changed (and in various degrees), and additional sets of experiments in which each possible combination of variables was changed (and in various degrees). Only then would we be able to judge the effectiveness of particular inputs in particular combinations and to answer such questions as: How important were the E program's efforts to augment patients' earnings, as contrasted, say, with the program's efforts to help patients with landlord, cooking, or social difficulties? Would better results (an excess of benefits over costs) have accompanied a reallocation of resources between these two types of efforts, or perhaps even the elimination of one or the other of them? A single experiment can only begin to provide data about the total production function for treating the mentally ill.

This conclusion leads to a generalization about all benefit-cost analyses: Benefit-cost analyses are inevitably incomplete in the sense that they compare only two (or, at most, a few) states of the world—typically with and without a certain project. Since a project is of a particular form, the analysis generally says little or nothing about the benefits and costs of any alternative form, duration, size, location, or other dimension. Occasionally, more than two alternative states are evaluated (for example, when the analysis of a possible dam project examines benefits and costs of various sizes for the dam). But the result is still examination of only a small portion of the total production function for a particular type of output. Whatever the findings, the possibility remains that some other resource combination would be more efficient than the one evaluated.

A final general issue applicable to all benefit-cost assessments is the usefulness of market prices in the valuation process. When prices of resources are determined in noncompetitive markets, those prices do not reflect the value of the resources in alternative uses. Thus, valuation of the costs of health care based on market prices will be sensitive to the degree of competitiveness of the markets involved. In addition, the market for health care often involves a substantial nonproprietary component. Seventy-six percent of psychiatric hospitals, for instance, are nonprofit, while 15 percent are operated by government. Nonprofit (38 percent) and public (16 percent) ownership also account for substantial numbers of homes for the mentally handicapped.[13] At this point we have no well-defined theory about the manner in which nonproprietary ownership affects price setting, but some authors have hypothesized that this too may cause prices to diverge from marginal social value.[14]

Even when actual and optimal prices diverge, however, the significance of the divergence depends on the variation across the alternative programs under consideration. If, for example, benefits and costs for two programs were being compared and these programs utilized inputs for which the divergences were essentially the same, then the relative efficiency of the two would not be affected by the distortions of prices. In general, however, this cannot be assumed; the analyst needs to examine and make judgments about the degree of competitiveness of the markets both for inputs and for outputs.

Regardless of the degree or character of competition, however, prices will, to some extent, reflect the purchasers' income (including wealth). Thus, any valuation of the benefits of health care based on willingness-to-pay as reflected by market prices will be sensitive to the income distribution. Though this criticism applies to all benefit-cost analysis, it may be particularly relevant to health care in that it is precisely because society believes that many who need health care are too poor to purchase it that social programs were established in this area.

As a result, the normative significance that should be attached to prices of inputs to and outputs from health care depends on the competitiveness of the markets and satisfaction with the distribution of income.

Benefits. Improving the health of patients is ostensibly the primary goal of any current treatment program. Such improvements may well increase the productivity and stability of patients and may bring "external" benefits to others; but to many people these results are secondary to the benefits of feeling better, that is, being more satisfied with life.

Measuring benefits of health programs is a challenging, critical problem. Is it any different, one might ask, from the problem of measuring benefits from any other good or service? Yes, I believe—and no. I will discuss the matter briefly, but it is surely a question deserving more research and debate.

At one level of analysis we can think of health services as one class among a large number of goods and services available to consumers. Knowing their own preferences, consumers observe the prices of all the available goods and services, and, given their incomes and wealth endowments, they choose how much to buy of each commodity, including health services.

One assumption embedded in the standard scenario, above, is that consumers can judge the quality of—that is, the benefits from— each good and service. In the case of many health services, and especially mental health services, that assumption is unjustified. First, people often are most in "need" of mental health services when they are least capable of making rational judgments. That is, even if a rational consumer would treat mental health services just like another commodity, a "seriously" mentally ill person would not generally be regarded as "rational." Willingness and ability to pay for mental health services would differ according to whether the person was or was not capable of making rational decisions.

Second, even a fully rational buyer of mental health services is often poorly informed about quality. One reason appeared in our earlier discussion of the counterfactual. Given the remarkable ability of the human body and mind to correct themselves, a mentally ill consumer would not necessarily improve or deteriorate, with or without treatment.

Third, and perhaps most important, particularly when "mental health" is involved, there is little consensus as to what that term means. One implication is that a consumer who is receiving some mental health services is in a position not merely of being poorly informed but of being unequally (asymmetrically) informed about the health service provider. The provider, acting as an agent for the patient, advises whether or not the patient should obtain or continue treatment. Thus, the provider could become involved in a conflict of interest, as a *principal* who might gain or lose income as a result of the advice. The efficiency and equity of the unregulated private market in mental health services should be studied, with special attention to the consequences of asymmetric information, "irrational" behavior, and the related agent-principal relationships.

It is clear that for a host of reasons measures must be developed of the degree of "success" or "failure" of mental health services. I suggest that success be defined in terms of achieving benefits. "Success" might be thought of in medical terms alone, but "benefits" suggests a wider range of dimensions.

In the Mendota study a number of dimensions or criteria were used for defining benefits. These included: (1) measures with an economic orientation—for example, earning power, employment stability, and evidence of financial planning (saving income and purchasing insurance); (2) clinical symptomatology measures developed by psychiatrists—for example, motor agitation, depressed mood, paranoid behavior; and (3) mental health status as judged by patients—that is, responses to the question, "How satisfied are you with life—friends, living situation, leisure activities?" with answers on a five-point scale ranging from one, "not at all satisfied," to five, "very much satisfied."

The potential for developing better measures seems to exist.[15] Some collaborative efforts between medical providers and economists seem desirable to develop measures that encompass both perspectives. If, as seems likely, multidimensional scales are appropriate, cross-disciplinary efforts will be required in order to move toward a comprehensive index that will, in turn, contribute to evaluating benefits within the benefit-cost framework.

Benefit-Cost Analysis versus Cost-Effectiveness Analyses. The fact that outputs and benefits of health programs are so difficult to define and measure has led to a search for evaluative approaches that do not require quantitative measurements of benefits. "Cost-effectiveness" analysis has emerged from this search.

A recent World Health Organization report defined cost-effectiveness analysis as "similar to CBA (cost-benefit-analysis) except that benefit, instead of being expressed in monetary terms, is expressed in results achieved, for example, number of lives saved or number of days free from [employee] absence."[16]

Thus, cost-effectiveness analysis involves comparison of program costs only—costs of alternative means of achieving a given (exogenously determined) level of outputs. The cost-effectiveness analyst leaves to other people—"policy makers"—the determination of what that level of output should be; the economic choice problem for the analyst is simply to find the lowest-cost means of producing that output. A cost-effectiveness analysis can be undertaken only when the technical experts understand enough about the production function to identify two or more input combinations that can produce the same output. Without an agreed-upon measure of output, however, that is impossible. Analysis would yield no evidence on the comparative costs of alternative programs for achieving the same output, only the costs of achieving different—and poorly understood—outputs.

It is technically feasible to compare the costs of alternative approaches to, say, the delivery of an hour of mental health services or the costs of alternative ways to find employment for the mentally ill. The same outputs (benefits), however, would not necessarily result from the alternative mechanisms. In fact, the Mendota experiment found that both benefits and costs differed across the programs that were compared.

The search for a way to sidestep the difficult tasks of defining and measuring benefits of improved mental health is misguided. Comparing the costs of programs with unmeasured and probably unequal benefits is not instructive for policy making.[17] At the very least, pains should be taken to identify differences in benefits when the analyst is comparing costs of obtaining seemingly similar benefits through different programs. Two programs that produce, for example, the same number of lives saved or days free from work-absence are not generally similar in other dimensions; the ages of the persons affected may differ or their post-program health status may differ (that is, one program may "save" lives and leave the persons in good health, while another program saves persons but leaves them injured and debilitated).

Aggregate Social Benefit Analysis. Just as one might focus on the costs of achieving unspecified outputs, so one might focus on the benefits of some unspecified inputs. In the earliest quantitative study by an economist in the mental health area, the author estimated the aggregate direct and indirect social costs of mental illness to the United States in a single year.[18] The same approach has also been used in other disease contexts such as polio and tuberculosis.[19]

In effect this approach estimates the benefits of some hypothetical program that totally eliminated mental illness. Since no such program exists in even an approximate form, and therefore no cost estimate can be developed, it is not clear that such aggregate benefit calculations are of value for public policy making.

Perhaps, however, it is technically feasible to undertake a program or programs that would cut the prevalence of mental illness by X percent. If it could be assumed that the aggregate social costs of mental illness would also drop by approximately X percent (or by some known function of X), then the aggregate figure would indeed be a useful basis for estimating the benefits from various mental health programs. Such an assumption does not, however, seem warranted. There has been little or no research attempting to identify general functional relationships between reductions in the prevalence or incidence of mental illness and magnitudes of reduced social costs.

Conclusion

Some form of benefit-cost analysis underlies every public action. The analysis may or may not be formal. It may or may not be quantitative. It may or may not distinguish between efficiency and equity dimensions. It may or may not measure up to the standards of economists. But in one fashion or another a judgment must be reached whether the advantages of the program outweigh the disadvantages. National expenditures on health are large and growing more rapidly than GNP. Careful scrutiny of the benefits and costs of existing and proposed health programs is thus greatly needed as a guide to intelligent decision making. Yet the potential for benefit-cost analysis should not be exaggerated. The best feasible benefit-cost analysis will measure variables with highly differing degrees of precision, including some with no objectively quantifiable value. This implies that benefit-cost analysis cannot be the sole basis for intelligent decision making. It can inform; it cannot substitute for judgment.

The next three chapters are case studies of benefit-cost analysis applied to different components of health care delivery. Chapter 5 deals with the effective prevention of poliomyelitis; chapter 6 considers community-based treatment of the mentally ill; chapter 7 concludes part two of this volume by analyzing the case of a new drug to treat duodenal ulcers.

Notes

1. The following are useful general discussions of benefit-cost analysis: Glen Cain and Robinson Hollister, "Evaluating Social Action Programs," in Robert Haveman and Julius Margolis, eds., *Public Expenditure and Policy Analysis* (Chicago: Rand-McNally, 1970); Robert Dorfman, "The Welfare Foundations of Cost-Benefit Analysis," *Economic Journal*, vol. 84 (1974), pp. 926-939; Robert Haveman and Burton A. Weisbrod, "Defining Benefits of Public Programs: Some Guidance for Policy Analysts," *Policy Analysis*, vol. 1 (1975), pp. 169-196; and the following textbooks: Edith Stokey and Richard Zeckhauser, *A Primer for Policy Analysis* (New York: W. W. Norton and Company, Inc., 1978); Robert Sugden and Alan Williams, *The Principles of Practical Cost Analysis* (New York: Oxford University Press, 1978).

2. The reader who wishes to examine the discount rate issue may wish to see the textbooks referred to in note 1, and also William Baumol, "On the Social Rate of Discount," *American Economic Review*, vol. 58 (1968), pp. 788-802; Martin Feldstein, "The Social Time Preference Discount Rate in Cost-Benefit Analysis," *Economic Journal*, vol. 74 (1964), pp. 360-379.

3. For a more detailed discussion of this issue see Murray Levin, "The Randomized Design Provides Circumstantial Evidence," *International Journal of Mental Health*, vol. 2 (1973), pp. 57-58.

4. See, for example, Finn Kamper-Jorgensen, "Scientific Methods in Long-Term Outcome Evaluation of Preventive Health Programs: A Critique of the Randomized Controlled Trial," *Scandinavian Journal of Social Medi-*

cine, Supplement 13, January 1977, pp. 81–91.

5. For an extended discussion of problems involved in controlled experimentation, see Jack Zusman and Raymond Bisonette, "The Case against Evaluation," *International Journal of Mental Health*, vol. 2 (1973), pp. 51-58.

6. Phillip May, "Cost-Efficiency of Mental Health Delivery Systems," *American Journal of Public Health*, vol. 60 (1970), pp. 2060-2067.

7. Burton A. Weisbrod, "Benefit-Cost Analysis of a Controlled Experiment: Treating the Mentally Ill," *Journal of Human Resources*, vol. 4 (1981), pp. 523-548; for a more complete report, see chapter 6.

8. One recent study refers to the stigma effect of having been treated for syphilis: Herbert Klarman, "Application of Cost-Benefit Analysis to the Health Services and the Special Case of Technologic Innovation," *International Journal of Health Services*, vol. 4 (1974), pp. 325-351.

9. For a statement of support for the basic needs view of social policy as compared with the generalized income-redistribution view, see Arnold Harberger, "On the Use of Distributional Weights in Social Cost-Benefit Analysis," *Journal of Political Economy, Supplement*, April 1978, pp. S.87-S.120.

10. Recognition of distributional effects of public programs suggests the possibility that some persons will actually be harmed by projects intended to be helpful. In such cases compensation may be desirable, both on equity grounds and to facilitate adoption of efficient programs. See Joseph Cordes and Burton A. Weisbrod, "Government Behavior in Response to Compensation Requirements," *Journal of Public Economics*, vol. 11 (1979), pp. 47-58; and Cordes and Weisbrod, "Compensating Losers from Economic Change When Lump-Sum Transfers Are Not Possible," mimeographed, Department of Economics, University of Wisconsin-Madison, 1982.

11. For a review of such problems see Richard Frank, "Cost-Benefit Analysis in Mental Health: A Review of the Literature," mimeographed, National Institute of Mental Health, Washington, D.C., 1979.

12. Various procedures for valuing human life are examined in Michael W. Jones-Lee, *The Value of Life: An Economic Analysis* (Chicago: University of Chicago Press, 1976), and Bryan C. Conley, "The Value of Human Life in the Demand for Safety: Extension and Reply," *American Economic Review*, vol. 68 (1978), pp. 717-720.

13. Current Population Reports, *1976 Survey of Institutionalized Persons*, Special Studies, Series P-23, no. 69 (June 1978).

14. Estelle James, "A Contribution to the Theory of the Nonprofit Organization," paper presented at the Conference on Institutional Choice, Madison, Wisconsin, October 23-25, 1979.

15. One writer has argued, however, that cost-benefit analysis is best applied to delivery systems rather than psychotherapy: Anthony Panzetta, "Cost-Benefit Studies in Psychiatry," *Comprehensive Psychiatry*, vol. 14 (1973), pp. 451-455.

16. World Health Organization (Copenhagen), *Cost/Benefit Analysis in Mental Health Services*, Report of a Conference, June 21-25, 1976,

ICP/MNH006 11, p. 9. See also the discussion by Finn Kamper-Jorgensen in that volume, pp. 31-43, on the distinction between cost-benefit and cost-effectiveness analysis.

17. Nonetheless, there have been a number of cost-effectiveness studies of mental health care. See, for example, Phillip May, "Cost Efficiency of Treatments for the Schizophrenic Patient," *American Journal of Psychiatry*, vol. 127 (1971), pp. 1382-1385; and Wilfred A. Cassell et al., "Comparing Costs of Hospital and Community Care," *Hospital and Community Psychiatry*, vol. 23 (1972), pp. 197-200.

18. Rashi Fein, *Economics of Mental Health* (New York: Basic Books, 1958).

19. Burton A. Weisbrod, *Economics of Public Health* (Philadelphia: University of Pennsylvania Press, 1961); Barbara Cooper and Dorothy Rice, "The Economic Cost of Illness Revisited," *Social Security Bulletin*, February 1976, pp. 21-36.

PART TWO

Benefits and Costs of Medical Research: Three Case Studies

5

Costs and Benefits of
Medical Research: A Case Study
of Poliomyelitis

Medical research has come to attract large and growing expenditures; the U.S. government alone spent more than $1.6 billion in 1969–1970, up from $45 million in 1959–1960 and from only $69 million a decade earlier.[1] Yet little is known about the economic efficiency of medical research—an activity which, having a substantial collective-consumption or public-good component, is financed in large part either by the federal government or by "nonprofit" organizations.

This paper examines costs and benefits of a particular medical research program that would generally be regarded as a medical "success"—the research which led to the development of vaccines (Salk and Sabin) against poliomyelitis. No attempt is made to generalize our findings to other medical research programs—either ongoing or prospective—although the paper does conclude with some brief comments on the possible wide applicability of the approach used here.

Why undertake a case study? What can be learned from it? First, if other case studies of medical research are undertaken, we may someday be able to develop generalizations as to the nature of the probability distribution of rates of return from various "types" of medical research and application programs. That is, theories may grow out of observations. Second, this case study will help to point

This paper originally appeared in the *Journal of Political Economy*, vol. 79, no. 3 (May/June 1971).

I benefited from the research assistance of Arden J. Lee and the late John Melder and also from comments by W. Lee Hansen, Alphonse Holtmann, Allen Kelley, Eugene Smolensky, and Leonard Weiss on an earlier draft of this paper. The research was supported by funds granted to the Institute for Research on Poverty pursuant to provisions of the Economic Opportunity Act of 1964 and also by the Health Economics Research Center, under a contract with the U.S. National Center for Health Services Research and Development. The conclusions are the sole responsibility of the author.

up the relationship between research and its application and the relevance of both to assessment of the social "profitability" of discovering new knowledge.

Third, the form in which the rate-of-return calculation is presented here can be thought of as constituting a checklist of items about which the informed public decision maker might seek information prior to making allocations of research funds among competing research programs.

The approach involves estimating the following: the time stream of research expenditures directed toward the disease (poliomyelitis); the time streams of a number of forms of benefits resulting from (or predicted to result from) the application of the knowledge generated by the research; and the cost of applying that knowledge. Finally, internal rates of return on the research expenditures are computed using several alternative sets of assumptions regarding costs and benefits.[2] In effect, we consider the rate of return that would have been obtained on polio research depending on which of a number of alternative states of events transpired and which alternative policy choices were (are) made subsequent to the technical success of the polio research program in 1957.

Evaluating benefits from medical research poses a problem not often encountered in other research. How should one evaluate a life saved or a lifetime of paralysis avoided? The complexity of the philosophical and empirical issues is clear. In this paper only a subset of the varied but elusive benefits from medical research is considered; these include (1) the increased production and (2) the reduced costs of treatment for persons who would have become ill or died from polio were it not for the successful research. Since total benefits are thus understated, our estimates of rates of return on costs will also be understated.

The internal rate of return on medical (polio) research—the rate which equates the time stream of research costs with the stream of benefits—is r in the denominator of the following expression:

$$\sum_{t=0}^{T} \frac{R_t - [B_t(N_t - W_t) - V_t]}{(1 + r)^t} = 0$$

where R is research costs, B is the benefit per case of the disease prevented (or the loss per case occurring), N is the number of cases occurring in the absence of a successful program of research and application, W is the number of cases occurring after a successful program of research and applications—so that $N - W$ is the number of cases prevented—V is the cost of applying the research findings, *t* is a particular year, and *T* is the terminal horizon year, the year beyond which the values of variables are asserted to be irrelevant (*T* could take on any value, including infinity).

The bracketed terms in the equation express the research benefits in year *t*, net of the cost, *V*, of applying the research knowledge. In the following sections, the operational form of each variable is discussed in the order in which it appears in the equation, with attention focused on the disease, poliomyelitis.

Research Costs

The nature of medical research is such that identifying an expenditure with a particular disease is frequently not easy. Expenditures on "basic" research—not directed at any disease—may contribute nonetheless to the development of an operational method for preventing some specific disease. And research aimed at a particular disease may produce results that are useful in dealing with some other disease. As a result, it is often not clear precisely what should be included in an estimate of the cost of research "on" a particular disease—for example, the research leading to the polio vaccines.

The conceptual problem is matched by the empirical problem of obtaining data. In table 5–1, column 2 shows the time series of amounts awarded for polio research, on the basis of information obtained by the Science Information Exchange (SIE). The data represent awards, not actual expenditures, and then only those research awards (grants and contracts) registered with the SIE by national granting agencies. The SIE series begins with 1946, and I have arbitrarily extended it back to 1930 in the interest of tolerable completeness. Because of the incompleteness of the SIE expenditure data and because of the necessarily arbitrary nature of the extrapolation, two alternative assumptions about the accuracy of the data are utilized in the calculations described below.

The research data in column 2 are in current dollars. In order to take account of price level changes, and in the absence of a truly satisfactory basis for doing so, I used the consumer price index (CPI) to adjust the expenditure estimates to the 1957 level of prices. The results appear in column 3.

Benefits per Case Prevented

In principle, "benefits" include *all* favorable effects in whatever forms are deemed relevant. As measured here, however, benefits from the prevention of polio are only the sum of: (1) the market value of pro-

TABLE 5–1

Estimated Awards for Poliomyelitis Research, 1930–1956
(thousands of dollars)

Year (1)	Current Dollars (2)	Price Adjusted (1957 = 100) (3)
1930	—	100
1931	—	200
1932	—	300
1933	—	300
1934	—	300
1935	—	300
1936	—	300
1937	—	300
1938	—	300
1939	—	300
1940	—	300
1941	—	100
1942	—	100
1943	—	100
1944	—	100
1945	—	100
1946	242	356
1947	492	631
1948	746	891
1949	1,513	1,823
1950	1,729	2,064
1951	2,609	2,883
1952	2,744	2,967
1953	2,022	2,170
1954	1,920	2,051
1955	2,176	2,332
1956	1,962	2,072

Source: Col. 2, Science Information Exchange; col. 3, for 1946-56, adjustments of data in col. 2 by CPI (1957 = 100); for 1930-45, author's estimates.

duction lost because of premature *mortality* due to polio; (2) the market value of production lost as a result of *morbidity*—illness and disability—caused by polio; and (3) the costs of resources devoted to *treatment* and *rehabilitation* of polio victims. The basic methodology by which each of these three components was estimated is described in detail in my *Economics of Public Health*[3] (hereinafter referred to as *EPH*) and will only be summarized briefly here. The present paper extends this earlier work, which dealt only with the benefit side, to an analysis in which the costs incurred to discover the effective vaccines and the costs of vaccinating people—applying the new knowledge—also are considered.

Mortality losses for people of specified ages had been estimated previously (in *EPH*) as the present value of expected future earnings,[4] utilizing 1951 earnings data and U.S. life tables for 1949–1951.[5] For women, the market earnings data were supplemented by estimates of the value of household services.[6] From these gross-loss figures were subtracted my estimates of the marginal consumption expenditures attributable to an incremental person in a household—the point being that mortality involves the loss of a consumer as well as a producer.[7] The resulting values of net future earnings were weighted by the actual reported number of deaths attributable to polio among males and females, by age, to obtain the estimated "premature mortality" loss per death from polio.[8]

Morbidity losses—those resulting from the temporary loss of a producer—were derived from the same age-specific and sex-specific earnings-productivity data used for the mortality-loss estimates, it being assumed that an average of one-fourth of a year of work time was lost per case because of temporary or permanent disability (*EPH*, table 9, and accompanying discussion). For the permanently and totally disabled, the entire remaining working lifetime was lost, but the overwhelming majority of cases produced little or no loss of work time—in part because the effects were very short-term and occurred among children.

Treatment losses are the third form of social cost of polio that had previously been estimated. Prevention of a disease makes treatment costs unnecessary, thereby liberating resources for alternative uses.[9] The range of treatment costs for polio victims has been great, running into many thousands of dollars when respiratory equipment was utilized, but for the large proportion of cases, which have been nonparalytic, these costs have been far smaller. Earlier, I estimated the mean at around $550 per case as of 1950.[10]

These three forms of losses were added together to give an estimated mean loss per case of $1,150—the estimate of the expected benefit per case prevented.[11] It is possible that a successful prevention program could bring about a significant change in the labor supply (and, hence, in the marginal productivity of labor) or in the demand for treatment; and in this case the $1,150 figure would be invalid. In the case of polio, however, the disease was not so widespread that substantial effects on factor supply or demand were likely to result from a successful prevention program.

Thus, it was assumed that for each case of polio prevented, a benefit of at least $1,150 resulted—"at least," because, as noted above, benefits in such important forms as reduced pain and suffering have not been considered. This estimated benefit per case prevented is derived from data for various years between 1949 and 1954, but because the data were largely from around 1950, the $1,150 figure was assumed to apply to that year. This figure has been adjusted to prices in 1957—the year of research "success," when the Sabin oral vaccine first became widely available—by the arbitrary use of the CPI, thereby producing a figure of $1,350 in 1957 prices. In some of the calculations described below, a productivity-growth adjustment was also made.

Number of Cases Prevented

We turn next to determination of the number of polio cases prevented. This requires estimation of the number of cases expected for each year following 1957, with and without the research success.

Expected Cases—No Research Success. During the period 1920–1956 the trend in reported cases of polio was upward, although there was substantial year-to-year variation.[12] Some of the "increase" was the result, simply, of improved reporting, and so the incidence rates for the later years should be given heavier weight in a forecast. The procedure actually used, therefore, was to calculate the mean rate for the ten years ending with 1956. This gave an average of some twenty-one new cases annually per 100,000 persons in the population. For the U.S. population in 1957—168 million—this produced an estimate of 36,000 new cases for each year after 1957, holding constant the size and age distribution of the population in that year.[13] Since the U.S. population is actually growing, and for reasons quite independent of the incidence of polio, the absolute number of polio cases would be expected to rise in the absence of a successful research program. The assumption of population constancy is relaxed, later, to assess the sensitivity of the rate of return to this assumption.

Expected Cases—Successful Research Program. Granted that in the absence of the research, 36,000 new cases of polio could be expected each year, it is necessary next to estimate the degree of success of the research. Here an important—if simple—point must be reiterated: knowledge without application is valueless. And since application of new knowledge is rarely costless, we can expect application of new knowledge to be less than complete and immediate. Polio vaccine illustrates this generalization. There are costs of producing and delivering vaccine, and there are implicit costs—in the form of time—for the individual taking it. Thus, we can expect the vaccine to be utilized by less than the entire vulnerable population under fifty, and, consequently, the number of new cases of polio may well not fall to zero.[14] In any event, we must take these application costs into account when we turn to the net benefits of the polio research effort, and this will be done below.

The number of new cases expected in a given year after the successful research is a function of the amount of resources devoted to vaccinating people over the previous forty to fifty years or so. The larger the expenditures on application of knowledge—that is, the more people vaccinated—the smaller the number of expected new cases.

In the procedure utilized in this paper, the number of cases expected after 1957 was assumed to equal zero, but alternative assumptions were employed regarding the number of persons who had to be vaccinated—and, hence, the total cost of vaccination—in order to produce this result. Alternative assumptions also were made regarding the cost per person vaccinated. Thus, in the equation above, $N_t - W_t$, the number of cases prevented, was assumed to equal 36,000, the number of cases expected in the absence of a successful research-vaccination program.

Application (Vaccination) Costs

Turning to the vaccination costs, V, it was assumed that to eliminate polio would have required (1) vaccinating the entire 1957 population under fifty,[15] (2) vaccinating all or, alternatively, none of the newborn children, assumed constant at the 1957 level of 4.25 million, and (3) incurring a vaccination cost per person of either $0.66 or $3.00 of direct cost plus an opportunity cost of time. The $0.66 figure assumes three "shots" (actually impregnated sugar cubes) at a cost of $0.22 each. This is an estimate of how low the cost might be if mass vaccination techniques were used.[16] It includes the purchase price of the drug, advertising costs, and my estimate of the implicit cost of the time donated by physicians, dentists, pharmacists, and others (utilizing 1959 income data for these occupations from the 1960 census). The total cost, so computed, was simply divided by the number of persons vaccinated to obtain the average cost estimate of $0.22 per shot, or $0.66 per person receiving the series of three. The $1.00 per shot alternative cost is a rough estimate of the charge made by private physicians (in 1957 prices).

Obtaining a vaccination also requires some of the time of the persons being vaccinated. In my calculations, the average opportunity cost of time per shot received was judged to be around $1.00 for adults and $0.50 for children. These figures are guesstimates. I assumed that about a half hour, including travel time, was required for each of the three shots at an opportunity cost of $2.00 per hour per adult. The lower figure for children (under eighteen) was based on the assumptions that, typically, a mother would take more than one child at a time, so that even if the mother herself was not also obtaining a vaccination, the opportunity cost to her of the time required would be well under the $1.00 per hour figure; in addition, in many instances, the vaccination would coincide with a physician visit for some other purpose, thus making the marginal time required rather modest.

Rates of Return

We can now relate the data on benefits and costs in order to obtain estimates of internal rates of return on polio research. Table 5–2 presents the rates of return under various assumptions about the variables, and with alternative time horizons.[17] Column 2 indicates the saving per case prevented (equivalent to the loss per case occurring, B in the rate-of-return equation above). In example I the assumption is made that the saving per case will remain constant over time at the 1957 level of $1,350. By contrast, examples II and III assume that the saving per case will increase over time. The reasoning is this: nearly half (actually $625) of the $1,350 figure consists of productivity (earnings) lost because of illness and premature mortality of polio victims. Since labor productivity may be expected to increase over time, a productivity-growth factor—of 3 percent per year—was applied in examples II and III to the labor-productivity portion of the $1,350 loss per case.[18]

As I discussed in a previous section, I estimated that an average of some 36,000 new cases of polio could be expected annually in the absence of a successful vaccine, assuming a constant population with constant age distribution. In making the estimates of the rate of return on polio research, I assumed, further, that the number of cases subsequent to 1957 would be negligible (strictly, zero) if everyone under age fifty were inoculated in 1957 and if, alternatively, (a) pessimistically, all newborn babies after 1957 would have to be inoculated in order to sustain the complete polio control (example III), or

TABLE 5–2

INTERNAL RATES OF RETURN ON POLIO RESEARCH UNDER
A VARIETY OF ALTERNATIVE ASSUMPTIONS

| Example (1) | Savings per Case Prevented (2) | Vaccination Costs (millions of dollars) | | Research Costs: Ratio of Actual to Reported (5) | Rate of Return (percent) | |
		In 1957 (3)	After 1957 (per year) (4)		1930–1980 (6)	1930–2200[a] (7)
I	Constant (at $1,350)	350	9	1	8.4	9.7
				5	5.1	7.0
		625	19	1	0.4	4.5
				5	−0.7	3.7
II	Growing	350	0	1	13.4	14.2
				5	9.0	10.4
		625	0	1	7.9	10.0
				5	5.8	8.4
III	Growing	350	9	1	11.7	12.9
				5	7.8	9.6
		625	19	1	4.5	8.1
				5	3.0	7.1

a. The rates in this column are also the asymptotic limits as the time horizon is extended.
SOURCE: Cols. 2-4, see discussion in text; col. 5, for "reported" data, see table 5-1 above; cols. 6-7, author's calculations.

(b) optimistically, no further inoculations of newborns would be required after 1957, the disease having been completely and permanently eliminated by the vaccination program in 1957 (example II). The truth, no doubt, is between these extremes; the object, however, is to assess the sensitivity of the rate-of-return estimate to a wide range of values of the variables.[19]

Columns 3 and 4 of table 5–2 reflect these and other alternative assumptions as to the cost of a completely successful vaccination program (V in the equation). The total vaccination costs in 1957 and, if necessary, thereafter are a function, of course, of the number of persons vaccinated and the cost per person. In each of the three examples in table 5–2 the assumption was made that the number of newborn children remained constant at the 1957 level of some 4.25 million. Later, this assumption is dropped.

Vaccination costs, as noted above, include the direct cost of producing and distributing the vaccine and also the opportunity cost of the time required to obtain the vaccination. In column 3 the cost of vaccinating the 1957 population under age fifty is shown for each of the three examples—first, under the low-cost assumption, $0.22 per shot plus opportunity cost, and second, under the high-cost assumption, $1.00 per shot plus opportunity cost. The respective total costs are $350 million and $625 million.

Column 4 is similar to column 3. It shows the estimated costs of vaccinating all newborn children in the years after 1957 under the low- and high-cost assumptions, which produce total costs of, respectively, $9 million and $19 million per year for the case of a constant number of newborns. (In example II, it is assumed that no post-1957 vaccinations are required.)

Column 5 reflects two alternative assumptions as to the accuracy of the data on polio research expenditures (awards) which appear in table 5–1. The rate-of-return estimates thus may be examined to see their sensitivity to substantial underestimates of the research-expenditure series. It is quite likely that the research series in table 5–1 understates the volume of resources entering polio research—in particular because it excludes expenditures by the pharmaceutical industry as well as expenditures on vaccine testing and on basic research that contributed to the eventual success of polio research efforts—but the degree of understatement remains a question. The rate-of-return estimates in table 5–2 have been made under the alternative assumptions that (a) the research-expenditure series in table 5–1 is essentially correct or (b) the true expenditures were five times as great as the figures in table 5–1.[20]

There is some possibility, however, that the polio research series in table 5–1 actually overstates expenditures devoted directly to polio research. For example, J. D. Watson comments that he had a Polio Foundation fellowship while doing research on the tobacco mosaic virus and on the DNA molecular structure[21]—research that ultimately led to the Nobel Prize for physiology and medicine in 1962 (shared with Francis H. D. Crick and Maurice H. F. Wilkens). It seems either that such expenditures should not be included fully in polio research costs or that the total benefits of polio research should be recognized as including external benefits—those extending beyond that specific disease. Either way, the result would be to raise the rates of return estimated in this paper.

Similarly, John F. Enders, Frederick C. Robbins, and Thomas H. Weller, who shared the Nobel Prize for physiology and medicine eight years earlier, in 1954, won it for discovering a simple method of growing polio virus in test tubes; yet their polio-related research had far more general value, for it "showed that viruses could be grown outside the body in tissues that they do not usually attack within the body."[22] Here again, we see that research produced a finding whose applicability was considerably wider than to polio alone.

Finally, a decision was required as to the time horizon relevant for the analysis. How far into the future should the savings from polio research be assumed to occur? Again, the procedure employed was intended to assess the implications of various choices of horizons. Five horizons were considered (1980, 1990, 2000, 2100, 2200), but the results for only two of them, 1980 and 2200, have been presented in table 5–2 (columns 6 and 7). There may be little justification for selecting a horizon as near as 1980; yet it may well be true that current vaccines will eventually yield to new strains of polio, and when that occurs the economic life of present vaccines will have ended.

The more distant the horizon, the larger the rate of return on polio research, although it is clear from table 5–2 that the rate-of-return estimates are not highly sensitive to the horizon choice. Among the dozens of cases considered—only some of which are reported in table 5–2–the extension of the horizon from the year 2100 for an additional 100 years never made a difference of more than one-tenth of 1 percent, and the extension from the year 2000 to 2100 seldom increased the rate of return by more than 1 percentage point. Considering the variety of alternative assumptions, the range of rates of return seems modest. Even extending the time horizon by 100 years or more beyond 1980 does not make a substantial difference in most of the cases examined. Generally speaking, the internal rates of return are within the range of 4–14 percent.

The "most likely" rate of return would seem to be about 11–12 percent. This conclusion was reached in the following way: (1) Since labor productivity (earnings) can be expected to continue to grow, examples II and III (table 5–2) seem to be more relevant than example I. (2) The most likely assumption regarding the need for post-1957 vaccinations is somewhere between the opposite extremes assumed in examples II and III, column 4, and so my choice of a rate of return will be bounded by these two examples. (3) Research expenditures reasonably ascribable to polio were probably less than three times as great as those reported in table 5–1 (although one certainly cannot be confident about this). (4) With respect to the social cost of applying the polio research knowledge, the low-cost-vaccination assumption seems to be preferable (for the high-cost assumption rests on an estimate of physician charges for individual vaccinations—charges which are likely to exceed the level of the marginal social cost that is possible when more efficient, mass inoculation techniques are used). A time horizon extending to the year 2100 or 2200—it makes virtually no difference which is selected—is reasonable.

These five judgments lead me to conclude that the most likely rate of return on polio research is between an upper bound of around 12 percent—the mean of the figures in column 7, fifth and sixth rows (example II)—and a lower bound of 11 percent—the mean of the figures in column 7 ninth and tenth rows (example III).[23]

Polio is a contagious disease, and, as a result, vaccinations produce external as well as internal benefits; because of this public-good nature of the commodity vaccination, our rate-of-return estimates would be even greater if the assumption were made that only a portion of the vulnerable population were vaccinated. The point is that, because of the external economies resulting from a vaccination, an increase in the proportion of population vaccinated will, up to some point, bring about a greater relative drop in disease incidence.[24] Beyond that point, diminishing external and internal benefits result from vaccination of additional persons.[25]

All of the rate-of-return estimates in table 5–2, however, may well be biased toward the low side—even with respect to the so-called economic consideration they are intended to reflect. For one thing, the benefits accruing outside the United States have been disregarded. (It is true, on the other hand, that research costs incurred outside the United States have also been ignored, but the sums involved are probably quite small.) For another, the risk aversion which doubtless characterizes most people's preferences has not been considered, benefits from reduced incidence of polio being estimated at their actuarial level.

Moreover, in order to be conservative, the productivity loss attributable to mortality from polio was taken to be net of the victim's expected individual consumption. Since death takes a consumer as well as a producer, this approach has some merit. Such a *net*-productivity view examines the losses from polio as they are seen by nonvictims, for whom the excess of a victim's productivity over his own consumption may be most relevant.

Alternatively, however, the point of view could be the entire society, including the victims who, of course, cannot be identified ex ante.[26] This would imply estimating mortality losses by *gross* productivity. Were this done, the mortality losses per case of polio would be increased by some 15 percent, but the total loss per case (including also treatment and morbidity losses) would rise by only some 5 percent.[27] Such an increased loss per case would raise the table 5–2 estimates of internal rates of return by only about one-half of 1 percent.

Another conservative assumption was that the number of newborn children would be constant at the level in 1957. If this number were assumed to increase at the rate of 2 percent per year—a figure somewhat larger than that which actually occurred in the United States during the decade 1950–1960[28]—the rate of return would rise by about 2 percentage points above the levels shown in table 5–2. Although the assumption of increase in the number of newborns raises vaccination costs, it also raises the number of cases of polio subsequently prevented.

Finally, but very significantly, some analysis of the importance of application costs is in order. The economic efficiency of research cannot properly be isolated from the costs of applying any new knowledge it generates. Expansion of knowledge and application of that knowledge are joint inputs, both of which are essential if benefits are to be obtained from any research. One implication of this point is that an efficient choice among alternative research strategies should take into account the costs of applying the research once it has become successful. A higher-cost research approach may be more efficient than a less costly one if the latter would entail greater application costs.[29]

To underscore the significance of application costs in the case of polio research, the rates of return summarized in table 5–2 have been reestimated under the assumption that successful research could be applied without cost, thus eliminating all vaccination costs. The results appear in table 5–3. The rates of return shown therein differ from those in table 5–2 for only one reason—the different assumptions regarding vaccination costs. (In the interest of expository simplicity, table 5–3 compares only some of the examples from table 5–2, specifically those involving the higher cost [$1 per shot] vaccination cost assumption. These appear in table 5–2, third, fourth, seventh, eighth, eleventh, and twelfth rows.)

Comparisons in table 5–3 between the rates of return in columns 3 and 4 and in columns 5 and 6 are striking. Whereas the assumptions of example I produced a rate of return of only 0.4 percent for the period 1930–1980, this would soar to 20 percent if there were no application (vaccination) costs. If there were no vaccination costs, it appears that, *ceteris paribus*, the internal rate of return on polio re-

TABLE 5–3

INTERNAL RATES OF RETURN ON POLIO RESEARCH, WITH AND WITHOUT VACCINATION COSTS

Example (1)	Research Costs: Ratio of Actual to Reported (2)	Rate of Return (percent)			
		1930–1980		1930–2200[a]	
		With vaccination costs (3)	Without vaccination costs (4)	With vaccination costs (5)	Without vaccination costs (6)
I	1	0.4	20.0	4.5	20.1
	5	−0.7	11.9	3.7	12.3
II	1	7.9	21.0	10.0	21.1
	5	5.8	13.2	8.4	13.6
III	1	4.5	21.0	8.1	21.1
	5	3.0	13.2	7.1	13.6

NOTE: The results in cols. 4 and 6 for examples II and III are identical. The reason is that these two examples differed in table 5-2 only with respect to their assumptions about post-1957 vaccination costs.

a. The rates in cols. 4 and 5 are also the asymptotic limits as the time horizon is extended.

SOURCE: Cols. 3 and 5, table 5-2 above; cols. 4 and 6, author's calculations.

search surely would have been satisfactory even by ordinary market standards—for the lowest rate of return shown in table 5–3 is 11.9 percent. If we disregard the costs of application, an erroneously high rate of return might have been assigned to the research effort alone. This would ignore the fundamental fact that research and its application are joint inputs to any disease control program.

This discussion of application costs grew out of the concern with returns from research, together with recognition of the relationship between research and application. The approach and the data presented here can also be used, however, to estimate the rate of return on programs to *apply* existing knowledge, taking as given the existence of the required knowledge and ignoring the sunk costs of research. In the case of polio, the research costs were small relative to estimated application costs, and so the expected rates of return, as of 1957, on a mass vaccination program are generally only 1–2 percentage points greater than the estimates in table 5–2, which reflect costs of research as well as vaccination.

Summary and Conclusion

The resources devoted to polio research in the United States have produced vaccines that are both safe and effective in preventing polio. The analysis in this paper shows that, except under the most extreme assumptions, this research is raising output and reducing treatment expenditures in amounts producing a rate of return on the research and application costs of at least 5 percent, or more probably 11–12 percent.

Because of the narrowness of the operational measure of benefits used in this paper, including its abstraction from the pain and anguish accompanying disease, there is little doubt that the real value of the medically successful polio research—and the price that buyers would pay for the vaccinations—is greater than what is estimated in this paper. The "value" of reduced illness and increased longevity is, one might guess, greater than simply the effects on earnings. In addition, even the more strictly financial benefits are probably understated, in part because of the disregard for the benefits occurring outside the United States.

Empirical findings as to the rate of return on polio research cannot be generalized to other medical research. The approach presented here, however, may have wider applicability.

In the case of some medical research programs, it may be possible to identify the disease or diseases that will be affected if and when the research is fruitful; the closer the research is to the "applied" end of the applied-basic spectrum, the greater the likelihood that such an identification can be made. When it can—when the output of medical research is expected to take the form of a reduction in the incidence, prevalence, or severity of one or more particular diseases—the variables in the internal-rate-of-return equation above constitute a checklist of items about which information should be sought by persons responsible for resource-allocation decisions: What is the expected cost of the research program in each period? If the research is "successful," what "benefits" will result in each future period (and with what probabilities) per case of the disease(s) prevented or made less severe? How many cases will be affected in each future period? What application costs, in each future period, will be required in order to realize these benefits from the medical research?

These questions will probably never be easily answered, and any answers will be uncertain. Uncertainty has not been considered explicitly in this paper; implicitly, however, variables have been evaluated in terms of expected values—a procedure that is not entirely satisfactory. Since it seems reasonable to assume that people are generally risk averters when disease is involved, the expected value of medical research will exceed the value of the expected benefits discussed above.

Recognition of the relationship between research and application points up some interesting facets of the "public good" problem and its connection with the question of allocative efficiency in the private sector. Knowledge resulting from (medical or other) research—for example, knowledge about means for preventing polio—has the characteristic of a public or collective-consumption good: its use by one person does not limit its availability to others. Thus, because of the familiar "free rider" problem, the production of medical research (knowledge) in the private market appears likely to be suboptimal. However, since the application of knowledge in some cases, such as polio, involves vaccinations or other procedures that are provided *individually*, exclusion of nonpayers is easily practiced. As a result, when investment in research and investment in the application of the resulting knowledge are considered jointly, the conclusion is that the private market may produce an optimal level of research.

This result, though possible, is by no means necessary. A priori, it is not clear to a private firm that if its research is successful the new knowledge will be such that it can be embodied in a salable commodity such as a vaccination. Even if it can, there is no assurance (except for patent laws) that competitors can be precluded from entering into the production of vaccines. Moreover, to the extent that any research is undertaken privately, we can expect it to emphasize exploration of techniques that lend themselves to low-cost exclusion of consumers—even if other techniques would be more efficient socially. The forms as well as the total "quantity" of research can be nonoptimal.

Another factor influencing the optimality of the private market provision of medical research and application is present when contagious diseases such as polio are involved. Since external benefits accompany the individual internal benefits of vaccination, the decentralized private market is likely to produce nonoptimal numbers of vaccinations; and since the expected profitability of research depends on the expected sales of vaccine, consumer decisions in the market for vaccinations will affect the profitability of research. On the one hand, the occurrence of external benefits tends to cause suboptimal purchase of vaccinations by consumers who disregard the benefits that their vaccinations bestow on others. On the other hand, if consumers also fail to adjust their decisions to the fact that they receive benefits from others who are being vaccinated, a superoptimal level of vaccination may result from individualistic behavior in the private market. The net effect on the vaccination market and, thus, on the research market seems unclear.

This paper has reported on a case study of costs and (certain) benefits of one medical research effort, polio. From the case study, however, we have also come to see how a benefit-cost analysis of medical research requires recognizing the interrelatedness of the research with procedures for applying the fruit of the research. Finally, we have seen that where collective-consumption goods, such as research knowledge, require the use of individual-consumption goods for their application, but where these individual goods produce real external economies, it may not be clear that the private market can be expected to behave inefficiently or, if it does, in which direction the deviation from optimality occurs.

Notes

1. Alfred M. Skolnick and Sophie R. Dales, "Social Welfare Expenditures, 1969–70," *Social Security Bulletin*, vol. 33 (December 1970), p. 4.

2. Internal rates of return have been estimated for various public expenditure programs. For example, for education see W. Lee Hansen, "Total and Private Rates of Return to Investment in Schooling," *Journal of Political Economy*, vol. 71 (April 1963), pp. 128-140. For water resources, see Robert Haveman, *Water Resource Investment and the Public Interest* (Nashville: Vanderbilt University Press, 1965), pp. 111-112. The return to only one governmental or nonprofit research effort has been estimated, on hybrid corn. See Zvi Griliches, "Research Cost and Social Returns: Hybrid Corn and Related Innovations," *Journal of Political Economy*, vol. 56 (October 1958), pp. 419-431. As far as I know, there has been no such estimation for a medical research program.

3. Burton A. Weisbrod, *Economics of Public Health* (Philadelphia: University of Pennsylvania Press, 1961), chapters 7 and 8 (hereinafter referred to as *EPH*).

4. Alternative discount rates of 10 and 5 percent were used, but the 10 percent calculations are utilized in the present paper. Except for the fact that the present-value estimates were already available from my earlier work (*EPH*), the undiscounted data would have been entered into the internal-rate-of-return formula. In addition, were it not for the fact that these estimates were already available, more recent data—for example, on earnings and life expectancies—would have been used.

5. *EPH*, tables 2 and 3. The assumption was made that age-specific and sex-specific incidence rates for other diseases are independent of those for polio. Thus, a reduction in the incidence of polio—as would result from a successful prevention program—was assumed to leave unchanged the incidence rates, morbidity, and mortality rates from other diseases.

6. Ibid., appendix 2.

7. For details of the estimation procedure see ibid., esp. pp. 33-34, tables 2, 6, and 12 and appendix 1.

8. Ibid., table 6.

9. It might be noted that a freeing of resources from treatment activities would produce no direct effect on the GNP, since treating the sick is regarded as a final output. Notwithstanding the absence of a change in measured GNP, it would seem clear that such a reallocation of resources—made possible by a successful disease-prevention program—would increase economic welfare.

10. *EPH*, p. 80.

11. Ibid., p. 90.

12. U.S. Department of Health, Education and Welfare, *Trends*, Washington, D.C., 1962, p. 17.

13. The age distribution is relevant because the incidence of polio is markedly age-specific. The incidence among persons over fifty has been virtually zero.

14. Since the number of cases prevented as well as the costs of prevention vary directly with the expenditures on applying knowledge, there is an economic optimum level of application; this may well involve less than complete vaccination of the population. In fact, as of 1970, 4.6 percent of all U.S. persons under age twenty are estimated to have had no polio vaccinations and an additional 15.2 percent had less than full protection—that is, less than three doses of either the oral or the injected vaccines. See U.S. Department of Health, Education and Welfare, *U.S. Immunization Survey—1969*, Washington, D.C., 1970, p. 13.

15. The Sabin vaccine provides lifetime protection.

16. The figure is derived from information provided by the Dane County (Madison), Wisconsin, "Sabin Oral Sunday" program. I have simply assumed that the costs of this program are representative of such programs generally.

17. The rate-of-return estimates are not, strictly, internal rates of return. The reason is that I utilized previously estimated data on benefits per case prevented, and these data included estimates of mortality loss which were, in turn, present values of expected future earnings, discounted at 10 percent (see n. 5 above and *EPH*, tables 2 and 3).

18. By adjusting the *treatment-cost* portion for price-level changes only, I have assumed implicitly that real costs of treatment would remain constant in the absence of a successful prevention program.

19. W. Lee Hansen has speculated that this procedure understates the expected rate of return because the poor are less likely to be vaccinated and their marginal productivity (as measured by earnings) is below average. Some recently available data confirm his prediction about vaccination. As of 1969, the proportions of the U.S. population aged one to twenty that were fully protected against polio by virtue of having at least three doses of either the oral or the injected vaccine were as follows: central cities poverty groups, 68.6 percent; central cities nonpoverty groups, 78.2 percent;

other poverty groups, 78 percent; other nonpoverty groups, 83.3 percent. The differences in percentages between "poverty" and "nonpoverty" (unfortunately not defined in the report) are significant at far better than the 0.01 level. See *U.S. Immunization Survey—1969*, p. 13 and p. 52, table B.

AUTHOR'S POSTNOTE (September 1982): The latest data on vaccinations that I have been able to discover are for 1977; at that time, the proportion of the population from birth through fourteen years of age that had at least three doses of polio vaccine were: central cities poverty groups, 47.8 percent; central cities nonpoverty groups, 60.4 percent. The difference became even greater than it had been in 1969. U.S. Department of Health, Education and Welfare, *U.S. Immunization Survey: 1977* (Atlanta: Center for Disease Control, 1978), p. 46.

20. A report by the American Medical Association states that the National Foundation spent some $41.3 million "for research related to vaccine development and for field trial studies." This is approximately twice as large as the total indicated in table 5-1. See American Medical Association, *Report of the Commission on the Cost of Medical Care*, vol. 3 (Chicago: American Medical Association, 1964), p. 45.

21. J. D. Watson, *The Double Helix* (New York: Atheneum, 1968), p. 132.

22. *World Book Encyclopedia*, 1965 edition, vol. 14, p. 347, and vol. 6, p. 223.

23. Although these estimates apply to the case of a medically successful research effort, not all expenditures on polio research contributed to the ultimate success of the Salk and Sabin vaccines. Thus, the estimated rates of return are, implicitly, weighted averages of the much larger rates of return on the "useful" lines of polio research and much smaller—perhaps even negative—rates of return on the less fruitful lines of polio research. Griliches notes the same circumstances with respect to the research on hybrid corn ("Research Cost and Social Returns," pp. 426-427).

24. To illustrate: 1969 incidence data (obviously unavailable in 1957) show that 95.4 percent of the U.S. population under age twenty had received some polio vaccination protection, and 80.2 percent had full protection (three doses of either the oral or the injected vaccine); but the number of reported new cases of polio has fallen by 99.9 percent and the number of deaths from polio has fallen by 100 percent! Cases decreased from between 15,000 and 57,000 per year during the 1950–1956 period to only 17 in 1969, and deaths dropped from 556 in 1956 to zero in 1969. U.S. Department of Health, Education, and Welfare, "Surveillance Summary: Poliomyelitis," *Morbidity and Mortality Weekly Report*, various issues.

AUTHOR'S POSTNOTE (September 1982): The most recent data available (for 1977) indicate eighteen reported cases of polio and zero deaths. Source: U.S. Department of Health, Education and Welfare, *Morbidity and Mortality Weekly Report: Annual Summary 1977* (Atlanta: Center for Disease Control, 1978), pp. 3,4. This report also cites data for years beginning with

1969, and the 1969 data vary somewhat from those reported previously in the "Surveillance Summary: Poliomyelitis." The 1977 report indicates twenty cases and thirteen deaths from polio in 1969, rather than the seventeen cases and zero deaths reported earlier. In any event the effects of the polio vaccine were clearly dramatic.

25. It does not follow, however, that a restricted vaccination program would necessarily be efficient, for the internal rate of return is not the appropriate maximand. For discussion of the latter point see, for example, W. S. Baumol, *Economic Theory and Operations Analysis*, 2d ed. (Englewood Cliffs, N.J.: Prentice-Hall, 1965), pp. 439-445.

26. Alternative points of view regarding definitions of "society" are discussed in *EPH*, pp. 35-36, n.7.

27. Measuring mortality losses by gross productivity adds only some 15 percent because of the manner in which consumption was estimated. Specifically, the concept was used of the *marginal* family consumption with respect to a change in family size; the marginal consumption, as expected, is considerably less than average consumption, the portion of aggregate income devoted to consumption. For additional discussion and computational details, see *EPH*, pp. 49-51, and appendix 1, pp. 100-113.

28. See *Statistical Abstracts of the U.S., 1964*. Since 1961, the absolute number of births has actually been decreasing.

29. Medically successful research that entails very great costs of application, for example, kidney dialysis machines, presents a most difficult social choice; either enormous costs must be incurred to provide sufficient machines, or decisions must be made as to which ill people will have access to the limited supply of machines and which ill people will die.

6

An Experiment in Treating the Mentally Ill: A Guide to Benefit-Cost Analysis

This chapter presents a new benefit-cost analysis of two alternative approaches for treating the mentally ill. With mental illness and its treatment becoming increasingly common and costly, and the already large public sector continuing to grow, the benefit-cost analysis presented here is important as a guide to resource allocation. Its purpose is to guide the prospective benefit-cost analyst working in any area, but especially in human services, in achieving a comprehensive view of the range of costs and benefits. This analysis extends beyond the area of mental illness to issues common to benefit-cost analysis in any area; for example, the usefulness of financial accounting data in cost estimation work, the relevance of distributional effects, and the recognition of "incommensurables" (costs and benefits that have not been translated into pecuniary terms).

Economic research on the evaluation of governmental programs has extended to a wide variety of activities,[1] and in recent years it

This research would not have been undertaken without the interest of Dr. Leonard Stein, who proposed undertaking an economic benefit-cost analysis in conjunction with the experiment that he and Dr. Mary Ann Test were designing at the Mendota Mental Health Institute, where they were, respectively, director and associate director of research. I thank them for their valuable help throughout this study. I also thank Margaret Helming, A. James Lee, and Olivia Mitchell for their significant contributions as research analysts, and Susan Feigenbaum, Steven LaValley, and Steven Verrill for their important research assistance. Helpful comments on an earlier draft of this paper were made by Janice Giesige. This study was supported by Grant 05-R-000009 from the National Institute of Mental Health, by the University of Wisconsin-Madison Health Economics Research Center, and by funds granted to the Institute for Research on Poverty at the University of Wisconsin-Madison by the Department of Health, Education, and Welfare pursuant to the provisions of the Economic Opportunity Act of 1964. An abridged version of this paper was published in the *Journal of Human Resources*, vol. 16, no. 4 (Fall 1981), pp. 523–48. This chapter appeared in Assaf Razin, Elhanan Helpman, and Efraim Sadka, eds., *Social Policy Evaluation: Health Education and Welfare* (will appear in 1983).

has increasingly used the methodology of controlled experimentation.[2] The study reported here is the first benefit-cost analysis of a controlled (random assignment) experiment in the mental health field. It compares, using an unusually wide variety of tangible and intangible forms of benefits and costs, a traditional hospital-based approach to treating the mentally ill with a nontraditional community-based approach, each to be described below.

From one point of view, this study is simply one more benefit-cost analysis of a social welfare program. As such, it interests those academicians and policy planners concerned with public policy issues as they affect the mentally ill. From another point of view, however, this is also a report on the use of a randomized experimental design for identifying the differential effects of policy alternatives. It is, then, a contribution to the growing literature assessing the strength and limitations of this approach in the real, as distinguished from the textbook, world.

This study illustrates yet another perspective: it is both important and feasible that economists and the experts of the pertinent field (here, mental health professionals) collaborate in designing and executing evaluative research. And finally, this study shows how to avoid, or at least reduce, errors in applied benefit-cost analysis and misunderstandings between analysts and users.

The use of benefit-cost analysis in public decision making has been criticized for reducing policy decisions to reliance on comparisons of dollar quantities only, while omitting effects not easily expressed in monetary terms or for which the assignment of monetary values can be made only arbitrarily.[3] If a benefit-cost analysis is performed properly, however, it will take into account as many as possible of the relevant variables, whether or not they can be either assigned money values or even quantified in nonmonetary terms. If such variables are made explicit, decision makers will be less likely to overlook them.

Another criticism of benefit-cost analysis is that it often seems to imply that decision makers can and should focus on economic efficiency; the assumption is that any adverse effects that create inequity can and will be neutralized by other public action (compensation).[4] The critical point, however, is that the incidence of spending decisions usually cannot be so easily offset, especially if the policies and projects under consideration would generate distributional effects outside the geographic and fiscal jurisdiction of the political decision-making unit. Such units, faced with very real budget constraints, have a legitimate interest in learning what expenditures they would have to make, as well as what nonmonetary costs and benefits would accrue to them, if a given program were to be adopted. Hence, decisions and the analyses on which they are based should take distributional effects into account, in addition to assessments of efficiency consequences.

Analytic Framework

Our study of the policy choice between two alternative approaches for treating the mentally ill poses in particularly stark terms the problems of what to measure and how to measure it. The very definition of mental illness is controversial, as are measures of the costs and benefits of its cure. Monetary values based on productivity gains and losses or on observed willingness to pay by patients and their families are, moreover, clearly incomplete because of patients' inability to make informed choices and because of external effects. The possibility that external effects (that is, the effects of one's actions on others) are sizable implies that assessment of costs and benefits must consider not merely the direct beneficiaries (patients in this case) but also a wide variety of other persons. Dispersion of costs and benefits beyond the group that constitutes the target is likely to be great in the mental health area, where the cost burdens of treatment fall not only upon individual patients, but also upon their families, as well as private philanthropists, insurers, and local, state, and federal government taxpayers. Similarly, the psychic costs of mental illness are borne not only by the ill person but also by family members and others with whom the ill person comes in contact.

Any benefit cost-analysis, therefore, in any project area, should carefully consider all consequences extending beyond the target group. Otherwise, a shift in the *form* of a cost or benefit may be misinterpreted or misestimated as a change in the *magnitude* of total costs or benefits.[5]

In the context of treating the mentally or physically ill, for example, a program that saves hospital resources by discharging patients from hospitals more quickly than usual will indeed reduce costs of hospitalization but will also shift costs to family members who care for the patient at home. Moreover, though hospitalized patients do not often become problems for the police, patients released under an early discharge program may well have contacts with law enforcement agencies and impose costs on the police system. In evaluating a proposed deinstitutionalization program, therefore, the benefit-cost analyst should not overlook the possibility that savings in real hospital costs could be offset by increases in law enforcement or other costs.

Any benefit-cost analysis should develop a comprehensive accounting framework. This minimizes the probability that when competing programs have benefits and costs that differ merely in form, they will not be mistaken for benefits and costs that differ in overall magnitude. In designing the benefit-cost analysis reported on here, we began with the development of just such a comprehensive framework. Even if it turned out that some forms of costs or benefits could not be measured, the accounting framework at least made the omissions explicit and thereby indicated the direction of probable estimation bias.

In general, the framework for any benefit-cost analysis (that is, for assessing the net present value of any project, V_j) may be summarized as follows:

$$V_j = \sum_{t=1}^{T} \frac{B_t - C_t}{(1 + r)^t}$$

where V_j = the value of project or activity j; B_t = benefits from the proposed program in year t; C_t = costs of the proposed program in year t; T = the planning horizon; and r = discount rate. If $V_j > 0$, the project is efficient.

The key problems, of course, are what to include in the benefits and costs, and which discount rate and planning horizon to use. In the case of the mental health experiment, data were obtained for only fourteen months; there is little need, therefore, to select a value for r, given that we can only observe results for a relatively short time interval. (Some comments will be made, however, about the consequences of the limited duration of the experiment.) Since the benefits and costs in this analysis are viewed from a social perspective, we are concerned with real benefits and costs, without respect to whether or not there are pecuniary exchanges.[6] (We shall see, however, that the distinction between real and pecuniary [transfer] changes can be difficult to make operational, even though the conceptual distinction is clear.)

As noted above, the external effects of treating the mentally ill are likely to be substantial. The patients' willingness to pay for treatment cannot be considered analogous to the demand for a private good, with the mentally ill alone demanding treatment. Other affected persons also demand treatment for the mentally ill, as do those who are affected only because they have interdependent utility functions that include the mental health state of others.[7] Even apart from these externalities, patients' own willingness to pay is not a satisfactory decision-making criterion, given that the mentally ill are not always able to make rational evaluations. In the quantitative estimates presented below, we attempt to measure the consequences of two treatment modes and thereby the difference in aggregate *social* willingness to pay for the two types of programs.[8]

Structuring the benefit-cost analysis is one step; employing the structure to measure the variables, once identified, is another. Some of the forms of benefits and costs will be satisfactorily measured in pecuniary units. For other forms, pecuniary measures will be available but controversial. For example, the number of lives saved or lost by some program might be presented in pecuniary terms, using one or another procedure;[9] alternatively, that number of lives might simply be presented, thereby leaving it to some decision maker to provide, explicitly or implicitly, the value weighting that will permit comparison. For still other forms of benefits or costs, there may be no available measure in pecuniary terms that is at all satisfactory.

This is not to say that any variable is, in principle, immeasurable. For some variables, however, either the conceptual foundation for measurement may be too weak to justify our presenting a pecuniary measure, or the costs of implementing the measure may be too high. For the same reasons, some variables will not be measured even in quantitative nonpecuniary terms; a qualitative (algebraic sign) indicator will sometimes be the optimal measure, for example, for the burdens on community members when the mentally ill live in residential areas. Finally, for some variables, the best that can be done will be no explicit measurement at all; a blank space or a question mark in a tabulation of benefits and costs is optimal.

In short, an optimal benefit-cost analysis—compared with an ideal one—measures variables with varying degrees of perfection. We expected the comprehensive benefit-cost framework for our mental health treatment programs (as for virtually any program or project in any field) to result in all of the following: some variables would be measured in pecuniary terms, some in quantitative but not pecuniary terms, some in qualitative terms, and some not at all. This discussion implies, therefore, that benefit-cost analysis cannot be the sole basis for intelligent decision making.

Experimental Design

Recent advances in pharmacology have revolutionized treatment of the mentally ill. This, together with changed social attitudes toward "warehousing" the mentally ill (institutionalizing them without treatment), has brought about sharp reductions both in the number of persons entering mental hospitals and the mean length of their stay. As table 6–1 shows, the number of patients in mental hospitals has

TABLE 6–1

Resident Patients and Admissions to State and County Mental Hospitals, United States, Selected Years, 1950–1977

Year	Resident Patients at End of Year	Admissions
1950	512,501	152,286
1955	558,922	178,003
1960	535,540	234,791
1965	475,202	316,664
1970	337,619	384,511
1974	215,573	374,554
1977	159,405	414,507

Sources: M. Kramer, "Psychiatric Services and the Changing Institutional Scene, 1950–1985," National Institute of Mental Health, *Analytical and Special Study Reports,* Series B, no 12, 1977; and *Statistical Abstract of the United States, 1981* (Washington, D.C.: U.S. Department of Commerce, Bureau of the Census, 1981), p. 117.

plummeted by some 60 percent from its peak of 559,000 in 1955 to 159,000 in 1977, and to an even lower level today. As the table also shows, however, the number of admissions has more than doubled during the period, from 153,000 to 415,000. With the increased turnover rate has come a phenomenon termed the "revolving door" syndrome—repeated admissions and discharges—which has led many experienced mental health professionals to wonder whether hospitalization might not actually be counterproductive for most patients.[10] If it is, then one or both of the following empirical hypotheses would hold:

Hypothesis 1: Patients treated in the hospital would have less favorable outcomes than would otherwise identical patients who were treated outside in a less dependency-creating environment.

Hypothesis 2: The long-run cost of treating the mentally ill outside the hospital would be lower than the cost of treating them in the type of hospital-based program currently in widespread use.

In the experiment to which we turn now, a comparison is made between the hospital-based treatment program in general use today, here called the control program (C), and a new community-based experimental program (E). The new E treatment approach actively supports persons in an outpatient setting.[11] Its essential characteristics are as follows: (1) Hospitalization is virtually eliminated. (2) Members of the staff work with patients in their neighborhoods, residences, and places of employment, providing support and teaching the coping skills necessary to maintain a satisfactory community adjustment. (3) The staff attempts to minimize the number of patients dropping out of treatment prematurely and to maximize their engagement in jobs and other aspects of responsible, independent community living.

The staff directed their efforts not only toward patients but also toward their families and the community setting. They held meetings with family members to help guide (or in many cases, to stop, at least temporarily) interactions when those were felt to be detrimental to the patient's adjustment. They also worked with community agencies, another effort felt to be critical if the E program was to succeed. According to Leonard I. Stein, M.D., and Mary Ann Test, Ph.D., developers of the program:

> Our major effort was to influence them to respond to patients in a manner that would promote responsible behavior rather than reinforce maladaptive modes of coping with stress. For example, if a patient's behavior was disruptive to other tenants in his apartment building, we would encourage the landlord to talk to the patient directly about his behavior and tell him he would be evicted if it continued. This is contrary to the community's usual response, which is to see to it that the patient's disruptive behavior leads to rehospitalization. That action implicitly gives the patient the message that he is not responsible for his behavior, teaches the patient a maladaptive mode of coping with stress and leads to a hardening of the chronic patient role.[12]

From an economic perspective, the E program is a system that confronts patients with the real social costs of their actions, compared with the traditional C-type approach, which largely does not. Under the C program, a mentally ill person who behaves in a socially unacceptable manner—on the job, in the roominghouse, in the community —is not punished, but, to the contrary, is typically rewarded with the protected and subsidized hospital environment that the individual prefers. Indeed, it is not uncommon for such persons intentionally to do things, including violating minor laws, so as to be sent back to the hospital. Thus, behavior that imposes external costs is actually rewarded!

Under the E program, by contrast, persons who impose costs on others are required to bear the consequences—the landlord's ire, losing a job, time in jail, etc. This is not to say that patients bear the full social cost; for example, they do not pay for the jail services.

An essential feature of the E program, however, is that patients are confronted more by the social costs of their actions than they are under the traditional C-type program. The underlying theory is that a mentally ill person behaves as a constrained utility-maximizer; the person's utility function may be warped, but he or she is seen as implicitly responding to relative prices, rewards, and punishments.

The experiment itself was conducted in the following manner. Subjects for both the experimental and control programs were all patients seeking admission to Mendota Mental Health Institute (MMHI) who (1) were residents of Dane County, Wisconsin (comprising the city of Madison and the surrounding area), (2) were between the ages of eighteen and sixty-two, and (3) had diagnoses other than severe organic brain syndrome or primary alcoholism. Beginning in October of 1972, 130 individuals were randomly assigned, in equal numbers, and continuing at the rate of four to six per month (two to three in each of the E and C groups), either to the E (community treatment) program or to the C program (the acute treatment ward in MMHI). The random assignment process resulted in a mix of E and C groups in which there were no statistically significant differences (0.05 level) between persons in the two groups in terms of age, sex distribution, marital status distribution, or time spent in psychiatric institutions (table 6–2).

The C program—the standard program at MMHI—consisted of progressive short-term, in-hospital treatment (generally lasting less than one month) plus traditional after-care provided by community mental health agencies. Patients who were assigned to the C group were screened immediately by a member of the hospital's acute treatment unit and were usually, though not always, admitted to the hospital. They remained a median of only seventeen days, but in many cases they soon returned to the hospital.

E subjects, by contrast, did not enter the hospital at all (except in rare cases when the need for intensive drug therapy or the risk of imminent danger to the life of the patient or others dictated some very brief hospitalization). Instead, they received the treatment approach of "community living" for fourteen months, after which they had no further contact with the experimental unit staff. Although no person in either the C or E program was part of the experiment for more than fourteen months, the experiment spanned a period of nearly three years, with patients entering and leaving each of the groups at the rate of two to three per month.

From the onset of the experiment, great efforts were made to avoid contamination of the study by "Hawthorne" effects. Such effects reflect the tendency of people who are knowingly involved in

TABLE 6-2

CHARACTERISTICS OF THE TWO TREATMENT GROUPS UPON ENTRY INTO THE EXPERIMENT

Characteristics	E Group (N = 65)	C Group (N = 65)
Sex		
Male	36	36
Female	29	29
Marital status		
Married	18	17
Divorced or separated	17	18
Never married	30	30
Age (years)		
Mean	31.5	30.5
Standard deviation	10.5	11.3
Prior time in psychiatric institutions (months)		
Mean	16.6	12.5
Standard deviation	31.0	28.9

SOURCE: Author.

an experiment to behave differently than they would otherwise, simply because they know they are involved in an experiment. There is no way to be certain that we were fully successful in avoiding such behavioral changes in patients, treatment staff, or research staff. Indeed, it was essential to the nature of the experiment that the professional staff and patients of the E program know that an experiment was under way.

Several facts lead to the belief, however, that Hawthorne effects are negligible in this case, and that any that are present are likely to bias behavior against, rather than in favor of, the E program: (1) *patients* in the E group knew that they were being treated in an unusual manner, but most were unhappy about being kept out of a hospital; if their attitudes, behavior, and recovery rates were affected at all (and it is not clear they were), it is likely to be because of these negative feelings; (2) *professional treatment staff* working with the E group had previously worked on a pilot community-based project; thus, the E-type program was not new to them; (3) *interviewers* who collected data about both the E and C groups were not involved in the clinical programs and had no vested interest in the outcome of the experiment; moreover, when interviewers met with research investigators, strict rules permitted talking only about research issues, not about patients; and (4) *families and community agencies* were often aware of the fact that some new treatment approach was being used and evaluated, but it is doubtful that they thought of themselves as being part of an experiment.

Data Collection. Data were collected for the sixty-five persons in each group at baseline (admission) and, for most variables, at four-month intervals during the subsequent year. To avoid any distorting effects caused by the adjustment of patients about to leave the E program, data from only the first twelve months (rather than fourteen) following each patient's admission were included in the analysis.[13]

In order to minimize sample attrition, great pains were taken to find out where former patients had relocated and to interview all of them. Research staff traveled as far as California to interview a patient who had moved there. Family members of a subsample of patients were also interviewed at the time of the patient's admission and again four months later. Information about patient contacts with various public and private agencies having been verified with the agencies involved, the economic research team met with staff of these agencies to ascertain the costs of the services provided.

Budget constraints limited the scope of the experiment in (1) the duration of the experiment, and (2) our ability to vary and control different combinations of variables. In any realistic (nonexperimental) application of the community-based program, patients would not likely be restricted to fourteen months of participation; thus, our experimental design permits only conjecture regarding whether the E program's success or its costs per patient year would be different if its duration were longer (or, for that matter, shorter).

As noted above, the E treatment approach differs not one but many simultaneous ways from the traditional C approach: (1) patients are not hospitalized; (2) patients live and work in the community; (3) people with whom patients are likely to come in contact are asked not to treat them differently from others because they are mental patients; (4) E group staff help patients find and retain jobs; (5) E group staff help patients to budget their money; (6) E group staff accompany patients to social activities; and (7) E group staff assist patients in a variety of other ways that are not available, or not available under the same conditions, to C group patients.

Because so many treatment variables are being altered simultaneously, any comparison of costs or benefits of the E or C programs can show only the overall net effect of altering the entire set of variables. As a theoretic ideal (abstracting from the costs of running multiple experiments), it would be desirable to run a set of experiments in which one treatment variable at a time was changed (and in various degrees), and additional sets of experiments in which each possible combination of variables was changed (and in various degrees). Only then would we be able to judge the effectiveness of particular inputs in particular combinations and to answer such questions as: how important were the E program's efforts to augment patients' earnings, compared with, say, the program's efforts to help patients with landlord, cooking, or social difficulties? Would better results (a larger excess of benefits over costs) have accompanied a reallocation of resources between these two types of efforts, or perhaps even the elimination of one or the other of these efforts? Our experiment can only begin to provide data about the total production function for treating the mentally ill.

This conclusion leads to a generalization about all benefit-cost analyses: *benefit-cost analyses are almost inevitably incomplete in the sense that they compare only two (or, at most, a few) states of the world—typically with and without some particular program.* Since a program is of a particular form, the analysis says little or nothing about the benefits and costs of any alternative form, duration, size, location, etc. Thus, just as the mental health experiment does not enable us to assess an alternative form of the E program (in which, say, job placement efforts were increased or reduced), so the typical benefit-cost analysis of a manpower training program, to take another example, fails to assess the consequences of having a different class size, job placement mechanism, or instructional system. Occasionally, more than two alternative states are evaluated (for example, when the analysis of a possible dam project examines benefits and costs of various sizes for the dam). The result, in any case, is examination of only a small portion of the total production function for a particular type of output. Whatever the findings, the possibility remains that some other resource combination would be more efficient than the one(s) evaluated.[14]

Estimating Costs and Benefits

Table 6–3 lists the forms of costs and benefits that it is desirable to measure. In the spirit of the discussion above, the table reflects the need for comprehensiveness of accounts, not ease or difficulty of measurement. With respect to measurement, however—the subject of this section—we may make the following generalizations:

- Although it is marginal costs and benefits that properly are of

TABLE 6–3
Types of Costs and Benefits

Costs	Benefits

1. Primary treatment
   MMHI
      Inpatient
      Outpatient
      Experimental center program
2. Secondary treatment
   Social service agencies
   Hospitals other than MMHI
   Sheltered workshops
   Other community agencies
   Private medical providers
3. Law enforcement and illegal activity
   Police
   Courts
   Probation and parole
   Property damage, human physical injury
4. Additional maintenance
   (food, housing, etc.)
5. Family burdens
   Property and wage losses
   Psychic losses
6. Burdens on other people
   (e.g., neighbors, co-workers)
7. Patient mortality
	1. Mental health
	2. Physical health
	3. Labor productivity
	4. Consumer decision-
	   making efficiency

SOURCE: Author.

concern in any benefit-cost analysis, the most readily available data will almost inevitably be averages.

• Averages derived from accounting records are frequently biased estimates of true social averages.

Both of these generalizations—and the dangers they suggest—apply to the mental health experiment. The estimates of benefits and costs presented here are mostly averages. Their use may be justified partly by their availability, but within the relevant range of variation, the long-run average and marginal costs (or benefits) may be roughly equal.

With regard to the use of organizations' accounting data, the estimates that follow are often derived from such records. In the case of the cost for treating patients at the MMHI, however (by far the largest cost component for the C group patients), major additions were made to the officially recorded cost data to reflect important components of long-run social costs not included in accounting costs (discussed below).[15] We turn now to a description of our efforts to measure each of the variables in table 6–3; our results, slightly reorganized, are in table 6–4.

Primary Treatment Costs. The daily cost of inpatient care at MMHI, as estimated by the state of Wisconsin, differed from the social costs of treatment in three respects, each of which led to an adjustment in the state-provided cost statistic: (1) the opportunity cost of the land on which the hospital is located had been disregarded; (2) the depreciation of the hospital buildings was based on historical cost rather than replacement cost; and (3) research carried out at MMHI was included in the per diem cost figure for the hospital. The per diem cost estimate by the state, approximately $70 in 1973, was adjusted upward to allow for an opportunity cost of 8 percent on the estimated value of the land and the depreciated replacement cost of the physical plant; it was adjusted slightly downward to account for research activities, which are not appropriately includable as treatment costs. The result was an increase to $100 in the MMHI per diem cost, our estimate of long-run marginal cost of treatment at that institution.

These adjustments made the MMHI treatment cost data more comparable with the experimental center cost data, for the latter also excluded research expenditures while including commercial rental payments for the center, and these payments presumably reflected a normal return on both the land and the depreciated replacement value of the physical structure.

C group patients also used facilities for outpatient treatment at MMHI. The average cost of such a contact was estimated by MMHI staff to average $10 per patient visit.

Calculating a long-run average cost for the E program is complicated by substantial variation in the rate of capacity utilization of its resources over the experimental period.[16] In order to make the estimate of average cost more closely approximate what the cost would be for a program in continuous, steady-state operation, we used data on the average cost (per patient per month) for the several months that the E program had a maximum number of patients.[17] This monthly figure was simply multiplied by twelve to obtain an estimate of annual cost per patient.

TABLE 6-4

Costs and Benefits per Patient, Experimental and Control Groups, for Twelve Months Following Admission to Experiment

Categories for Which Monetary Estimates Have Been Made	Control Group (C) (1)	Experimental Group (E) (2)	E − C (3)
Costs			
1. Direct treatment costs			
MMHI			
Inpatient	$3,096	$ 94	−$3,022**
Outpatient	42	0	−42**
Experimental center program	0	4,704	4,704†
Total	$3,138	$4,798	$1,660†
2. Indirect treatment costs			
Social service agencies[a]	$1,744	$ 646	−$1,098**
Hospitals other than MMHI			
Sheltered workshops (Madison Opportunity Center, Inc., and Goodwill Industries)	91	870	779**
Other community agencies			
Dane County Mental Health Center	55	50	−5
Dane County Social Services	41	25	−16**
State Dept. of Vocational Rehabilitation	185	209	24[b]
Visiting Nurse Service	0	23	23**
State Employment Service	4	3	−1*

Private medical providers	22[c]	12	−10[a]
Total	$2,142	$1,838	−$ 304†
3. Law enforcement costs			
Overnights in jail	$ 159	$ 152	−$ 7[a]
Court contacts	17	12	−5[a]
Probation and parole	189	143	−46
Police contacts	44	43	−1[a]
Total	$ 409	$ 350	−$ 59†
4. Maintenance costs	$1,487	$1,035	−$ 452
5. Family burden costs (lost earnings due to the patient)	$ 120	$ 72	−$ 48[e,f]
Total costs for which monetary estimates have been made	$7,296	$8,093	$ 797†
Other costs			
6. Other family burden costs			
Number of families reporting physical illness due to the patient	25%	14%	−11%[e]
Percentage of family members experiencing emotional strain due to the patient	48%	25%	−23%[e,i]
7. Burdens on other people (e.g., neighbors, co-workers)	?	?	?
8. Illegal activity costs			
Total number of arrests	1.0	0.8	−0.2[a]
Total number of arrests for felony	0.2	0.2	0.0[a]
9. Patient mortality costs (percentage dying during the year)			
Suicide	1.5	1.5	0
Natural causes	0	4.6	4.6

(Table continues)

TABLE 6-4 (continued)

Categories for Which Monetary Estimates Have Been Made	Control Group (C) (1)	Experimental Group (E) (2)	E − C (3)
Benefits			
1. Earnings[h]	$1,136	$2,169	$1,033**[d]
From competitive employment	1,136	2,169	1,033**[d]
From sheltered workshops	32	195	163**[d]
Total	$1,168	$2,364	$1,196†
Other benefits			
2. Labor market behavior			
Days of competitive employment per year	77	127	50[d]
Days of sheltered employment per year	10	89	79[d]
Percentage of days missed from job	3%	7%	4%[d]
Number of beneficial job changes	2	3	1[g]
Number of detrimental job changes	2	2	0[g]
3. Improved consumer decision making			
Insurance expenditures	$ 33	$ 56	$ 23[d]
Percentage of group having savings accounts	27%	34%	7%
Summary			
Valued benefits	$1,168	$2,364	$1,196
Valued costs	7,296	8,093	797
Net (benefits − costs)	−$6,128	−$5,729	$ 399†

* Significant at the 0.10 level.

** Significant at the 0.05 level.

† Significance not tested; the number is a sum of means.

a. These data were derived from agency or patient reports on the number of contacts; patient reports were used only when it was not possible, or was excessively costly, to obtain the relevant information from the agency. Estimates on contacts were obtained from the agency.

b. Data from the Department of Vocational Rehabilitation (DVR) were available only for the twenty-eight-month study period as a whole, which included the follow-up period after the experiment. The per patient costs are 12/28, or 43 percent of the twenty-eight-month data, reflecting average cost for one year. The figures reflect some double counting because much of the DVR expenditures go for payments to other agencies that are included in the table in section 2 under costs. We have been able to account for, and to exclude, DVR payments to the sheltered workshops but not, for example, to hospitals. The $24 difference is biased upward by the omission of counselling expenses attributable only to C group members.

c. These figures include fees for physicians, psychologists, and nurses, but exclude any associated laboratory fees.

d. These data are derived from patient reports and as such are subject to misreporting. Patient reports were used only when it was not possible (or was excessively costly) to obtain the relevant information from an independent source. In some cases, when an interviewer with information on all patients were sometimes able to provide it on this spot-check basis.

e. These figures are derived from interviews conducted four months after admission with twenty-two families of E group patients and eighteen families of C group patients (34 percent of the E group, 27 percent of the C group). The other families were not interviewed because: (1) they lived outside of Dane County (23 percent of each group); (2) the subject or the family refused to cooperate (12 percent of the E group, 22 percent of the C group); or (3) the relative could not be contacted (31 percent of the E group, 28 percent of the C group). The questionnaire examined the families' experience in the two weeks preceding the interview only, and, with some trepidation, these figures are inflated to an annual average. The reduced sample size and the single interview yielded data which must be interpreted with caution.

f. These figures were derived by multiplying the number of days family members missed work because of the patient by a daily wage of $24 (or $3 an hour).

g. Our judgments, based on examination of patient reports.

h. Earnings do not include value of fringe benefits, if there were any.

i. Interviewers' assessments.

Secondary Treatment Costs. Secondary treatment includes the wide range of medical and related helping services provided by various agencies, institutions, and professions, and made available to both groups of patients outside of their respective primary treatment facilities. The category thus includes hospitals and psychiatric institutions other than MMHI, halfway houses, sheltered workshops, visiting nurses, counseling and educational services, etc.

Patient interviews provided initial data on the number of service units received or contacts with secondary providers; these were verified by all major local providers, but not—for reasons of cost—by small local providers (for example, doctors) or out-of-town providers, with the exception of other state-run hospitals in Wisconsin.

Measures of the costs of treatment by the numerous secondary providers were short of the ideal of long-run average social cost—and not simply (or even primarily) because of input price distortions. Even in those few instances where we had access to cost data—and most providers were unwilling to provide it—time and staff constraints dictated that we simply accept the providers' own estimates of the costs of servicing the C and E group subjects. Another generalization about benefit-cost analyses can be made: *In any benefit-cost analysis in which cost information is derived from records of firms or other institutions, budgetary constraints together with organizations' reluctance to provide access to their financial records usually lead to the use of imperfect and biased cost data.*

Law Enforcement Costs. Another form of social costs that may vary with the treatment mode is law enforcement. We were able to obtain data from patient interviews on the number of police and court contacts, the number of nights spent in jail, and the number of contacts with probation and parole officers. Reported contacts with the Madison Police Department and the Dane County Sheriff's Office were verified, but those with other departments were not. The costs per contact or per overnight were obtained by methods essentially the same as those used for secondary treatment costs.[18]

External Costs Caused by Patients' Illnesses. Patients interact with other persons in a wide range of settings. Although we do not have information on all such interactions, we have examined two categories of individuals for whom these external (to the patient) costs are likely to be particularly great: members of the patients' immediate families, and other people who have suffered because of illegal—or at least disruptive—behavior on the part of patients. We obtained data on the burdens imposed on people in these two categories from interviews with patient families at baseline (time of admission to the E or C programs) and after four months, as well as from records of courts and law enforcement agencies.

Clearly, however, these measures are imperfect, and there are difficult problems in assigning monetary values. Many of the burdens can be translated into costs only by essentially arbitrary methods. What, for instance, is the cost of worry or of the disruption of a person's normal routine? In principle, the willingness of the affected persons to avoid these costs is measurable, but we were unable to develop such monetary values. Our limited ability to deal with external costs suggests another generalization: *even when relevant forms of costs are not quantified in monetary terms, they can at least be enumerated explicitly.*

In the interviews with family members (at baseline and after four months), families were asked whether or not they had experienced work or school absences, disruption of domestic or social routines, trouble with neighbors, or stress-related physical ailments as a result of the patient's illness.[19] They were also asked whether the patient's illness had forced them to purchase services formerly provided by the patient, whether they had paid for psychiatric treatment or medication received by the patient, and whether they had given cash or large noncash gifts to the patient. With this information the interviewer rated each family as suffering a severe, moderate, or mild burden (or no burden) from the patient's illness.

Patient Maintenance Costs. On the one hand, it can be argued that maintenance is simply a requirement of living, thus is not a function of mental health status, and so should be excluded from the table. On the other hand, the E program encouraged, as a deliberate aspect of its treatment methodology, independent living arrangements; therefore, the resulting higher level of maintenance costs is a real cost of this treatment mode.[20] In principle, we should include as real costs only the incremental maintenance costs attributable to the E program. In practice, however, it is not only extraordinarily difficult to identify these additional costs, it is not even clear that this increment is positive. If the E program were more effective, for example, it might well result in more efficient consumption behavior and hence lower consumption/maintenance costs (expenditures) than would otherwise have been incurred.[21]

Improved Mental Health of the Patient. Improving the mental health of patients is ostensibly the primary goal of any current treatment program. Such improvement may well increase the productivity and stability of patients as consumers and may bring external benefits in the forms discussed earlier, but to many people all of this is secondary to the benefits of patients' feeling better, that is, more satisfied with life.[22]

These effects are difficult to value in monetary terms, even conceptually. For ordinary goods and services, a patient's behavior might reveal a willingness to pay. With regard to the mentally ill, however, it is not clear either what normative meaning should be attached to the person's stated willingness to pay for better health or what kinds of inferences about that willingness should be made from any observed behavior.

In the quantitative work presented below there are no pecuniary values for the state of a subject's mental health per se or for changes in that state. This is one of the variables for which quantitative but nonpecuniary indicators seem most appropriate. Three such indicators are used: (1) various objective measures of quality of life, such as the number of leisure-time social groups the subject reported having attended in the month preceding the interview (at four, eight, and twelve months); (2) a trained interviewer's judgment of the presence or absence of various symptoms of mental illness, plus an overall assessment of "global illness"; and (3) the subject's own assessment of how satisfied he or she is with life (living situation, friends, food, work, etc.). Each of these is described in the next section, where the empirical results are presented.

Improved Productive Behavior of Patients. One potential benefit of any treatment program for mentally ill adults is an improvement in a patient's lifetime ability to function as an economic producer. A full accounting for increased productivity would encompass not only increases in marginal productivity in the organized market but also increases in nonmarket productivity, such as unpaid work around the home and increased investment in human capital (perhaps via education) which can be expected to increase the present value of productivity in the future.

Conceptually, we want to measure any increase in productive *potential* that is attributable to treatment. A reallocation of patients' time between work and nonwork is not necessarily a benefit of effective treatment. Thus, to anticipate a finding reported below, if the E patients worked more than did the C patients, the resulting differential in earnings would not necessarily constitute a benefit.

There are two reasons for believing, however, that an increase in the earnings of mentally ill persons as a result of treatment should be regarded as a social benefit, even if such an increase was a result of increased hours of work (and decreased hours of "leisure"). First, for the mentally ill, the opportunity cost of work time at the margin —that is, the reservation wage—might be close to zero. This is not implausible, considering the difficulty that the mentally ill have in gaining employment for the desired number of hours per week. Indeed, given their emotional problems, the negative psychological feelings associated with leisure (where one lacks the company of other people in the work setting and lacks social approval for work) might well be such that the marginal value of leisure is even negative.[23] Second, persons with mental illness typically have difficulty in retaining a job. Thus, if one treatment mode results in a greater increase in earnings, this might reasonably be interpreted as a differential program benefit whether the added earnings occurred because of an increased hourly rate of pay or an increase in the amount of time worked.

Wages paid in competitive employment are a reasonable proxy for the marginal product of the individual's labor, even though the absence of perfectly competitive markets means that market wages do not usually equal the value of the worker's marginal product. Wage determination in sheltered workshops, however, is not a directly market-determined process. Workers (patients) do produce goods and services in workshop programs and are paid wages.[24] Their productivity, however, is often far below that of persons competitively employed to produce a similar product and, indeed, the patients' pay is often far below the minimum wage. State and federal laws require that wages in sheltered workshops be determined by comparison with the wage rates and productivity prevailing in the competitive market. If a worker's productivity is, say, 60 percent of that of competitively employed individuals doing the same type of work, then the worker's pay must be 60 percent of the going wage for that job. It appears that the sheltered workshops in the Madison, Wisconsin, area do make a serious effort to pay the mandated wage, which approximates the value of the marginal product of the work.

Data on work experience and earnings were obtained from the quarterly interviews with patients. As a rough check on the accuracy of responses, social security wage records were examined (in the 92 percent of cases for which records could be obtained). Information on sheltered workshop employment and earnings was provided by the workshops themselves.

Housework or child care work for one's own family typically involves no pecuniary exchange, which makes the evaluation of such work difficult. Despite our attempts, in the end we were unable to obtain a useful measure of the quantity or value of household work.

Participation in an educational or training program is an investment activity to the extent that it increases productive potential and hence the present value of future earning capacity. Given the brief duration of our experiment (one year), it would be hazardous to project the value of any education or training that a subject might have obtained during the single year when, for at least part of the year, the person was acutely ill. No data were obtained for the effect of each treatment mode on this human-capital investment variable.

Increased Work Stability. Wages, either actual or imputed, are not the only useful measure by which the effects on productivity of the two treatment modes should be assessed. Work stability is another. Current stability provides some evidence of future stability, and hence can serve as an indicator of expected earnings beyond the period of the experiment. Thus, we attempted to measure the differences in the job stability of the C and E group patients.

One such measure of productive stability is "absenteeism"—the percentage of days on which the patient was expected to be at a job but was absent. A second measure of stability is the number of "beneficial" and "detrimental" job changes made by the patient. Any statistically significant differences in the number of beneficial changes (for example, moving to a job with a higher wage rate) and detrimental changes (for example, being fired) can reasonably be considered evidence of differences in the effectiveness of the two treatment programs.

Improved Consumer Decision Making. One potential benefit of a successful treatment program is that individuals improve their ability to manage their finances. Indicators of such benefits, let alone monetary values for them, are difficult to devise. We present below information on two indicators, both of which are, at most, only suggestive. One is the subject's expenditures on insurance, reflecting the patient's attention to the future and its uncertainties. The psychiatrist and psychologist directing the experiment believe that, within limits, increased attention to the future is a sign of improved mental health. It should be noted, however, that though expenditures on insurance may be an *indicator* of improved health and, hence, of social benefits, such expenditures do not themselves constitute a *measure* of benefits that can simply be added to benefits in the form of, say, increased earnings.

The same is true for a second indicator of more efficient consumer behavior for the mentally ill—behavior with regard to saving. Again the psychiatrists' interpretation is that more saving, within limits, reflects increased, and healthy, concern for the future. As an operational matter, we were able to obtain useful data only on whether the subject did or did not have a savings account; neither the size of the account nor the presence of savings in other forms could be ascertained.

These two indicators are far from satisfactory. They are included primarily as illustrations of a class of benefit variables that is relevant but easily overlooked—more efficient use of available resources. By including them, the benefit-cost analyst underscores to the policy maker the necessity to make a judgment about their importance.

The relevant period for analysis is the period over which all of the benefits are realized and all the costs incurred, perhaps a lifetime or even longer if mentally ill parents affect the mental or physical health of their children. It is likely that for any treatment program the time pattern of costs and of benefits are not the same, costs being concentrated at the onset of the treatment program and benefits being spread out over a longer interval. Moreover, the time patterns may well differ among alternative treatment modes. As a result, a one-year analysis—even if it were complete—may provide a misleading picture of lifetime benefit-cost relationships, both for any given treatment mode and across treatment modes. A treatment program should be viewed and evaluated as an investment yielding returns (pecuniary and nonpecuniary) through time. Thus, the ideal benefit-cost analysis would identify the time patterns of net benefits as well as a discount rate.[25]

Figure 6–1 sketches a plausible time pattern for the differentials between programs in total benefits and in total costs. It portrays costs that, during the course of the first four months of treatment, are increasingly greater for the average E program patient. The extra cost of the E program, $C_E - C_C$, then diminishes, while the excess of benefits of the E program over the C program increases, so that by the end of the twelfth month, the higher cost of the E program is offset by its extra benefits.

Findings

In this section we present estimates of the variables for which measures were described in the previous section. As the reader will expect by now, some measures will not be in dollar form. All benefits and costs shown in table 6–3 are listed again in table 6–4, with either dollar quantities, nonmonetary numerical estimates, or simply question marks. The question marks are particularly notable. They highlight variables that, though relevant to comprehensive benefit-cost

FIGURE 6-1

HYPOTHETICAL NET BENEFIT AND COST STREAMS
FOR TWO TREATMENT MODES

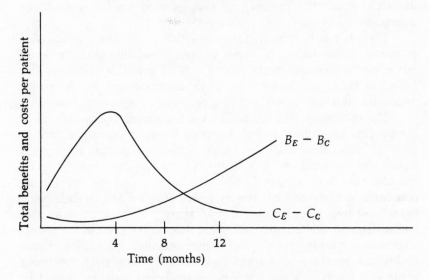

analysis, have not been quantified. Such variables are often omitted from benefit-cost analyses, but here their inclusion, if only by using question marks, serves to underscore the fact that quantitative estimates—monetary or other—have not been made. They are thus an explicit reminder of the need for policy makers to judge their importance.

Tables 6-5 and 6-6 are companions to table 6-4. Table 6-5 shows the real quantity units which lie behind the pecuniary data in table 6-4; when multiplied by the respective prices, these quantities yielded the dollar amounts shown in table 6-4. Table 6-6 gives some detail about the mental health measures listed in table 6-4.

It bears repeating that this benefit-cost analysis deals with only two alternatives, the status quo (C program) and the particular constellation of community-based efforts (E program). The question is whether the E program is "better"—on either cost or benefit grounds or both—than the C program, not whether the E program (or the C program) is better than any of a large number of other alternative programs.

Costs. Several findings are apparent from table 6-4: (1) Average total dollar costs are of substantial magnitude—$7,300–$8,100 per patient year—whichever treatment approach is used, and only about half of

TABLE 6–5

Quantities of Services or Resources Utilized per Patient, Experimental and Control Groups, for Twelve Months Following Admission to Experiment

	Group	
Costs	C	E
1. Direct treatment costs		
MMHI		
Inpatient days	31.4	3.0
Outpatient visits	6.1	0.0
2. Indirect treatment costs		
Social service agencies		
Hospitals other than MMHI	n.a.	n.a.
Sheltered workshops days	5.6	52.3
Other community agencies		
Dane County Mental Health Services Board (contacts)	3.8	6.8
Dane County Social Services (contacts)	2.8	1.8
State Employment Service (days)	0.5	0.2
Private medical providers: contacts	1.9	1.3
3. Law enforcement costs		
Overnights in jail	15.9	15.7
Court contacts	0.3	0.2
Probation and parole (occurrences)	2.2	1.5
Police contacts (arrests)	0.5	0.7

Note: n.a. = not available.
Source: Author.

the total is in the form of primary treatment costs. (2) Average total dollar costs of mental illness including its treatment are some 10 percent higher for the E program than for the C program. (3) As anticipated, the forms of costs are quite different for the two treatment approaches. The E program entails, for example, 50 percent *greater* direct treatment costs—$4,798 per E program patient compared with $3,138 per C program patient. Similarly, while there is only about a 15 percent difference (in favor of the E group) in total indirect treatment costs, some components of indirect costs show a much greater difference. The "other hospital" component of E program costs is

TABLE 6–6
Mental Health Indicators for E and C Subjects

Indicator	Findings
Symptomatology[a]	
At end of:	
4 months	E group was significantly (0.05 level or better) less symptomatic on 4 of the 13 measures (including global illness); on the other 9, no significant differences.
8 months	E group was significantly (0.05 or better) less symptomatic on 4 of the 13 measures (including global illness); on the other 9, no significant differences.
12 months	E group was significantly (0.05 or better) less symptomatic on 7 of the 13 measures (including global illness); on the other 6, no significant differences.
Social relationships[b]	
At end of:	
4 months	E group had significantly (0.05) more (2.1 vs. 0.7).
8 months	E group had significantly (0.05) more (1.7 vs. 0.8).
12 months	E group had significantly (0.05) more (1.9 vs. 0.6).
Patient satisfaction with life[c]	
At end of:	
4 months	No significant difference between E and C.
8 months	No significant difference between E and C.
12 months	E group significantly (0.05) higher mean score.

a. Thirteen items were considered, consisting of the following twelve symptoms plus an overall independent assessment of "global illness": depressed mood, suicidal trends, anxiety or fear, expression of anger, social withdrawal, motor agitation, motor retardation, paranoid behavior, hallucinations, thought disorder, hyperactivity-elation, and physical complaints.
b. Number of social groups attended in the last month.
c. On a 5-point scale from 1, "not at all satisfied" (with friends, living situation, leisure activities) to 5, "very much satisfied."
Source: Author.

110

some 60 percent smaller than that of the C program, about $650 per patient for the E group. Sheltered workshop costs are nine times as large annually for the E group—$870 versus $91. Maintenance costs are 40 percent greater for the C group program patient—$1,487 versus $1,035 per patient year.

Recall the hypothesis that the E patients would have more contacts with the law because they spent more time in the community. Table 6–4 shows that the opposite was the case, whether the measure is number of arrests, number of felony arrests, or the associated law enforcement costs. E group patients, by our measures, also imposed fewer burdens on their families, although the differences are not statistically significant.

Finally, it should be noted that there is not a statistically significant difference in the number of deaths from natural causes, and no difference at all in the number of suicides. Table 6–4 intentionally stops short of placing a monetary value on lost human lives. Estimates of such values have been made elsewhere, but both the conceptual foundations of the various approaches and the resulting estimates vary a great deal.[26] As a result it seemed best to refrain from introducing explicit valuations of life into the table.

Benefits. Treatment of the mentally ill can be viewed as having the goals of helping the patients to "feel better" and to be more productive members of society. Operational measures of achievement of these goals are required for a benefit-cost analysis. Tables 6–4 and 6–6 show four types of benefit measures.

1. *Earnings and labor market behavior.* The discussion in the section on the improved productive behavior of patients pointed out that though earnings from increased work are in most contexts an overestimate of net welfare benefits, for the mentally ill this may not be the case. The marginal disutility of work for the mentally ill, who are frequently unable to obtain or to retain a job, may well be close to zero. It may even be negative; that is, the satisfaction from working in a socially approved way may well exceed the pecuniary rewards.

Table 6–4 shows that E group patients showed substantially better labor market performance as measured by earnings. They averaged more than twice the earnings of control group members, and almost all of the excess was from competitive employment rather than from sheltered workshops. The greater earnings were realized despite the E group's higher (but not significantly different) absenteeism rate— 7 percent compared with 3 percent for the C group—and, in general, workers were not paid for days missed.

2. *Consumer decision making.* Do the treatment programs differ in their ability to aid patients to use their resources more efficiently, that is, to maximize their utility subject to the budget constraint? The conventional assumption that consumers are successful as utility maximizers can reasonably be questioned for the mentally ill. We can view their behavior as either the failure to maximize utility or their maximization of an "inappropriate" utility function (one they would not have but for their illness); in either case, however, treatment can help patients to be more effective decision makers.

Data problems were particularly serious in this area. We were able to estimate insurance expenditures and the presence or absence of a savings account, both of which reflect forward-thinking behavior, as discussed in the preceding section. But there were not significant differences between the programs, and in any case, these measures leave much to be desired. The differences that were found, however, favor the E program.

3. *Mental health status as judged by outside observers.* There is no single measure or indicator of mental health. One approach adopted in this experiment called for a trained observer to meet with patients and report on the presence or absence of various adverse symptoms. In the first section of table 6-6 are the findings that the E group averaged fewer symptoms at the four- and eight-month interviews and still fewer at the twelve-month interview. These findings are even more striking when it is realized that the E group was actually more symptomatic at the time of admission (a fact not reported in the table).

The second section of table 6-6 presents another indicator of mental health status—frequency of social relationships. Since the mentally ill tend to withdraw from social contacts, more frequent contacts are interpreted as favorable. E group members consistently had more social relationships than did C group patients. (The difference did not grow, however, through the year of treatment.)

4. *Mental health status as judged by patients.* The third section of table 6-6 shows that though the E and C patients reported no significant difference in "satisfaction with life" after four and eight months, the E group experienced significantly greater satisfaction by the end of month twelve.

All of these findings indicate that E patients, who were spending a significantly greater proportion of their time in the community, were becoming better adjusted socially and were experiencing improvement in their quality of life—measured in various ways and from differing perspectives—as compared with the C group. This leads to several observations about these quantitative findings:

• Our initial concern about the danger of mistaking a shift in the *form* of cost for a change in the *level* of cost proved to be well founded. If we had neglected, for example, to examine the costs of providing sheltered workshop services, we would have found that average total costs were virtually identical for the two programs, whereas, because the workshops were used far more by the E patients, the E program was 10 percent more costly in total. And if we had limited our attention to hospitals in the county, rather than extending it to other "out of town" hospitals, we would have underestimated the C program per patient cost by $808 per year while underestimating the E program cost by only $264 per year.

• The enhanced earnings of the E group patients apparently led to a reduction in the amount of maintenance costs borne by others. The $1,196 of increased patient earnings per year under the E program was accompanied by a decrease of $452 in maintenance costs. Assuming equivalent living standards for the two groups, the added earnings of the E group were, in effect, "taxed" at a 38 percent marginal rate.

• The somewhat greater costs of the E program appeared to bring an even greater increase in benefits. Tables 6–4 and 6–6 show that the E program, while more costly in real terms, has added benefits in the form of labor market earnings alone that exceed the added costs. When the mental health benefits, as described in table 6–6, are considered, the net advantage to the E program grows further.

Summing up the quantitative findings we find that the experimental programs (1) cost an additional $800 per patient year, but in return increased productivity (as measured by earnings) by some $1,200; (2) showed evidence of enhancing the planning and decision-making skills of patients (insurance and savings behavior); (3) decreased mental illness symptoms of patients; (4) increased a sense of satisfaction with life for patients. The evidence suggests that the community-based E approach would justify the added cost, assuming that the benefit-cost relationship estimated in a single-year experiment would hold over time.[27]

The Distribution of Cost Burdens

Benefit-cost analyses typically are regarded as efforts to determine how efficiently the resources of proposed governmental projects or programs are allocated.[28] Questions of who bears the costs and who reaps the benefits are usually not examined, reflecting economists' unwillingness to make comparisons of personal utility. As a matter of positive economics, however, our ability to predict governmental behavior surely would be enhanced if we understood better the distributional consequences of governmental programs.[29]

There are many ways to view distributional effects. The data in table 6–4 can serve as a starting point from which to identify who receives the benefits and who bears the costs. Patients receive the earnings, less some percentage that is taxed, and patients also receive any increased satisfaction with life. Family members benefit from any reduced burdens. Taxpayers gain (or lose) from decreases (or increases) in utilization of publicly provided services.

Table 6–7 was developed to shed light on the distributional effects of choosing one treatment approach rather than another. It shows the initial incidence of monetary costs for both programs. (The possibility of shifting is not examined here.) The dollar costs shown in table 6–4 have been allocated according to the funding sources for each cost item; since many of the individual costs in the earlier table were funded by several different sources, numbers appearing in table 6–7 have a complex relationship with those in table 6–4.

Columns 1 and 2 show how our cost estimate of $7,296 per patient year for the C program is distributed among the four classes of governmental and private groups. It is noteworthy that although *state* mental hospitals are frequently thought of as the basic locus of treatment (and hence of costs), only 37 percent of total monetized costs are borne by the state under the prevailing C-type program. As was pointed out above, current treatment of the mentally ill does not usually involve long-term custodial care, and so the average patient in the C program is out of a hospital the vast majority of the time even in the year following an acute episode. When the person is outside the hospital, he or she is likely to be using a wide variety of mental health and related services that are financed either by private donors or by local and federal governments.

Columns 3–6 of table 6–7 reflect two alternative assumptions as to the distribution of costs if the experimental approach were adopted. Columns 3 and 4 show the distribution under the assumption that the E program was run by the Dane County Mental Health Center and was financed from various sources in the same proportion as the center is now financed; columns 5 and 6 assume the program would be run by MMHI and financed as that institution is now financed.[30]

A priori, I expected to find that the division of monetary costs (the only costs dealt with in table 6–7) of the E and C programs would differ substantially among federal, state, and local taxpayers, and private persons, and this has indeed been the case. The traditional treatment approach (C program) for the mentally ill has placed heavy emphasis on hospitalization—and mental hospitals have been financed

TABLE 6–7

INCIDENCE OF FIRST-YEAR COSTS FOR CONTROL
AND EXPERIMENTAL PROGRAMS

	Control Program		Experimental Program[a]		Experimental Program[b]	
	Dollars (1)	Percent (2)	Dollars (3)	Percent (4)	Dollars (5)	Percent (6)
Government						
Federal	1,731	24	1,240	15	1,142	14
State	2,707	37	4,802	59	3,771	47
Local	1,563	21	767	10	2,191	27
Private[c]	1,269	17	1,127	14	980	12
N.E.C.[d]	26	0	157	2	9	0
Total	7,296	99	8,093	100	8,093	100

a. This distribution assumes the Experimental Center Program costs are distributed as the Dane County Mental Health Center costs.

b. This distribution assumes the Experimental Center Program costs are distributed as the Mendota Mental Health Institute costs.

c. These figures include private individuals' contributions, support by private nongovernmental agencies such as the Salvation Army, and commercial insurance.

d. Not elsewhere classified; this category includes private medical provider costs and miscellaneous "other" costs.

SOURCE: This table is derived from table 6-4; totals may differ slightly because of rounding.

largely by state governments. At the time our experiment was begun, the governor of Wisconsin was pressing the legislature to close one of the two state mental hospitals in order to reduce the state budget. Although this would surely be a cost-reducing action in the first instance, it was not clear that state fiscal burdens would be reduced in the aggregate. The mentally ill might impose increased cost burdens on other institutions receiving some state finance (for example, prisons and sheltered workshops). It was even less clear how any savings to the state would compare with added costs imposed on other levels of governments and on nongovernmental persons and institutions.

Pressure by various governors and state legislators to close state mental hospitals appears to reflect a somewhat mistaken view regarding the importance of state funds in financing the care and treatment of the mentally ill. As columns 3–6 in table 6-7 show, by contrast with columns 1–2, the shifting of treatment from the currently pre-dominant C-type program to the community-based E-type program would *increase*, not decrease, both the percentage and the absolute dollar-cost burden on state taxpayers under either of the two assumptions regarding how the Experimental Center costs would be shared. (There is no basis for saying what would have happened to either costs or benefits if the state mental hospital had been closed, or if the patients in the E program had been kept out of the hospital but had not been provided with the resources for the E program; neither of these counterfactuals was part of the experimental design.)

Table 6–7 also shows that the experimental program, while being about 10 percent more costly than the control program, has the effect —under the assumptions regarding Experimental Center cost distributions of either columns 3–4 or columns 5–6—of reducing dollar cost burdens on private donors and on federal taxpayers. Tax burdens on state taxpayers, by contrast, are sharply higher under the community-based E program, whichever finance method is used. Burdens on local taxpayers either rise or fall, depending on which of our two assumptions is made as to who would finance the Experimental Center costs. Table 6–7 deals with the costs for which monetary values appear in table 6–4; the distribution of nonmonetary costs, however, is also relevant to a full assessment of the welfare effects of the two treatment approaches.

Disaggregating Patients by Diagnosis

The overall average comparison of E and C groups, as in table 6–4, can mask systematic variation in costs and benefits for particular "types" of patients. Patients are, after all, inputs to the mental health production process. Thus, the relative costs and the relative benefits of the E and C production processes may vary among patients whose mental illnesses differ. If this were the case, it would hold that the benefit-cost relationship for treating some types of mental illness would favor the E program and for other types it would favor the C program technology.

Table 6–8 shows the benefits and costs in the manner portrayed in table 6–4, but for each of the three diagnostic categories (determined at time of admission) for which the sample size was meaningful: schizophrenics, other psychotics (nonschizophrenic), and persons with personality disorders (PD). The direct treatment cost of the E patients could not be estimated separately by diagnostic category; therefore the tables show the same cost figure.

116

The contrasts in both benefits and costs for persons with each type of mental illness is striking. Direct treatment costs for the C patients averaged $1,964 per PD patient, but were more than twice as large, $4,276, per schizophrenic patient. Law enforcement costs for E patients ranged from $75 per year for nonschizophrenic psychotic patients, $332 for schizophrenics, to $944 for PD patients. Moreover, while the law enforcement cost for nonschizophrenic psychotics was four times as large under the C program as under the E ($307 compared with $75), the relative costs were reversed for the PD group. The C program patients were associated with considerably smaller costs—$572 compared with $944. (The differences are not statistically significant at the 0.05 level, but this is not surprising, given the sample sizes.)

When the "total costs for which monetary estimates have been made" are examined across diagnostic classes, we again find notable differences. The costs of the two treatment technologies as applied to nonschizophrenic psychotics differ by only a little over $100. For schizophrenics, average costs of E and C programs differ by less than $300, with the C costs being greater. For PD patients, however, the difference was nearly $2,600 per patient year.

Variation on the benefit side is just as noteworthy. Table 6–4 had shown that E patients earned twice the approximately $1,100 earned by C patients. Now we see that earnings within the C group ranged from $725 for nonschizophrenic psychotic patients to nearly $1,400 for those with personality disorders. And E group earnings ranged from $1,319 for PD patients to $3,113 for nonschizophrenic psychotics. The differential earnings between the E and C treatment approaches was some $2,400 for nonschizophrenic psychotic patients, in favor of the E program, but it was only $70 for PD patients and in favor of the C group.

The disaggregated findings in table 6–8 are important not simply because they disclose variation around the means in table 6–4, but because the diagnostic categories are discernible at baseline. Thus, patients could be sorted out at the time an acute problem develops, with treatment—E or C—depending on diagnosis. The data, imperfect as they are, suggest that the E program is "preferred"—in terms of monetized benefits and costs only—for schizophrenics and other psychotics but not for PD patients.

Another Look at Program Effectiveness

The fact that E and C group patients were randomly assigned does not preclude the possibility that systematic differences in relevant vari-

TABLE 6-8
Costs and Benefits per Patient, Experimental and Control Groups, for the Twelve Months Following Admission to Experiment

Categories for Which Estimates Have Been Made	Schizophrenics			Personality Disorders			Nonschizophrenic Psychotics		
	C (N=26)	E (N=33)	E − C	C (N=16)	E (N=11)	E − C	C (N=8)	E (N=9)	E − C
Costs									
Primary treatment									
Mendota Mental Health Center	$4,276	$ 98	−$4,178**	$1,964	$ 3	−$1,961**	$3,033	$ 89	−$2,944**
Experimental center program	0	4,704	4,704†	0	4,704	4,704	0	4,704	4,704
Total primary treatment costs	$4,276	$4,802	$ 526†	$1,964	$4,704	$2,743	$3,033	$4,793	$1,760
Secondary treatment									
Social service agencies									
Other hospitals (Non-MMHI)	1,764	474	−1,290	2,231	1,577	−654	1,831	675	−1,156
Sheltered workshops	73	1,073	1,000**	135	176	41	56	496	440
Other community agencies	121	243	122	154	140	−14	114	232	118
Private medical providers	37	22	−15	217	184	−33	236	20	−216
Total secondary treatment costs	$1,995	$1,812	−$ 183	$2,737	$2,077	−$ 660	$2,237	$1,423	−$ 814
Law enforcement	453	332	−121	572	944	372	307	75	−232
Maintenance	1,453	1,020	−463	1,607	1,266	−341	1,278	671	−607
Family burden costs (lost earnings)	26	0	−26	26	489	463	0	0	0

Total costs for which monetary estimates have been made	$8,233	$7,966	−$ 267	$6,906	$9,480	$2,577	$6,855	$6,962	$ 107
Other family burden costs Percentage of families reporting physical illness due to the patient	54%	21%	−33%	38%	27%	−11%	75%	56%	−19%
Illegal activity costs (number of times charged with a misdemeanor or felony)	0.1	1.1	1.0	.6	.5	−.1	.6	.0	−.6

Benefits

Benefits for which monetary estimates have been made Earnings									
From competitive employment	$ 945	$1,477	$ 532	$1,345	$1,293	−$ 52	$ 664	$2,870	$2,206*
From sheltered workshops	24	271	247**	46	26	−20	61	243	182
Total benefits for which monetary estimates have been made	$ 969	$1,748	$ 779	$1,391	$1,319	−$ 72	$ 725	$3,113	$2,388

Summary

Valued benefits minus costs									
Valued benefits	$ 969	$1,748	$ 779	$1,391	$1,319	−$ 72	$ 725	$3,113	$2,388
Valued costs	8,233	7,966	−267	6,906	9,483	2,577	6,855	6,962	107
Net (benefits − costs)	−$7,264	−$6,218	$1,046	−$5,515	−$8,164	−$2,649	−$6,130	−$3,849	$2,281

** Significant at 0.05 level.
† Significance not tested, as the number is a sum of means.

ables will affect the experimental results. In this section a regression approach is used as another way to examine the overall effectiveness of the E and C treatment technologies. First we reexamine the effect of treatment mode on patient earnings and then on clinical ratings.

Effects of Treatment Technique on Earnings. Equation 1 presents the findings from a regression (OLS) of patient earnings in dollar per year $(T.E.)$, on four background variables—age, years of schooling, dummies for marital status (1 if married) and sex (1 if female)—as well as on a dummy variable (E/C), for the treatment group (1 if E).

$$T.E. = -804 + 13\,Age + 182\,Yr\,Ed + 585\,Marr - 1{,}322\,Fe$$
$$\quad\;\; (0.66) \quad (0.61) \quad\;\; (2.27) \quad\quad (1.29) \quad\quad (3.26)$$
$$+\,768\,E/C \tag{1}$$
$$\quad (1.93)$$
$$R^2 = .19 \qquad N = 101 \qquad \text{(t-statistics in parentheses)}$$

Recall that table 6–4 had shown that E patients averaged more than \$1,100 higher earnings than C patients during the twelve-month period; but equation 1 estimates the difference attributable to the E program at \$768. Apparently, the random assignment process produced some systematic differences across groups.

Even more striking is the effect, in equation 2, of controlling for patients' earnings in the year prior to participation in the experiment (in either the E or C program). When this variable, $YLag$, is added, the apparent effect of the E program falls further (from \$768 to \$507), its statistical significance declines, and the value of R^2 rises to .54, from .19 in equation 1.

$$T.E. = -1{,}719 - 2\,Age + 176\,Yr\,Ed - 87\,Marr + 115\,Fe$$
$$\quad\quad (1.85) \quad (0.13) \quad\;\; (2.90) \quad\quad (0.25) \quad\;\; (0.33)$$
$$+\,66\,YLag + 507\,E/C \tag{2}$$
$$\;\; (8.53) \quad\quad (1.68)$$
$$R^2 = .54$$

The $YLag$ variable was added to control for the possibility—which seems to be the actuality—that patients in the E program happened by chance to have been more productive prior to admission; in that case they might well have had greater post-admission earnings even if the E program were *less* effective than the C program.

A comparison of equations 1 and 2 also shows that adding $YLag$ changed drastically the coefficient on the sex variable, Fe, from a negative and highly significant \$1,322 to a positive but not significant

$115. The importance and significance of marital status also dropped sharply, and the sign changed.

Next, in equation 3, I added dummy variables for type of patient's illness, following the reasoning of the preceding section. (Dummies were added for only the two diagnoses with the largest sample sizes —schizophrenics and personality disorders. Between them they accounted for about two-thirds of the patients in both the E and C groups.)

$$T.E. = -1{,}399 \underset{(0.31)}{-5\,Age} \underset{(2.55)}{+157\,Yr\,Ed} \underset{(0.43)}{-164\,Marr} \underset{(0.18)}{+63\,Fe} \underset{(8.25)}{+64\,Lag}$$

$$\underset{(0.02)}{+8S} \underset{(0.39)}{+217PD} \underset{(2.32)}{+1{,}237\,E/C} \underset{(1.14)}{-807S^{*}E} \underset{(2.00)}{-1{,}647PD^{*}E}$$

$$R^2 = .57 \tag{3}$$

where S and PD refer to schizophrenic and personality disorder diagnoses, and $S^{*}E$ and $PD^{*}E$ refer to interactions of each diagnosis with participation in the E treatment program. (Complete data on the variables used in equations 1 through 3 were available for only 101 of the total of 130 patients. I am aware of no reason to expect selection bias.)

The contrast with the results in table 6–8 are marked. Table 6–8 showed that schizophrenic patients in the E program received $779 more earnings per year than did their C group counterparts. Equation 3 implies, however, that, *ceteris paribus*, a schizophrenic patient in the E program can expect only $430 more than a schizophrenic patient in the C group ($1,237 less $807). For a patient with a diagnosis of PD, the results are even more striking. The E program appears to be less productive than the C program, at least in terms of earnings; participation in the E program is associated with *lower* earnings than could be expected by a PD patient treated in the more traditional C mode— $1,237 less $1,647, or —$410. Table 6–8 also had shown lower earnings for the E patients, but only $72.

The regression analysis advanced the preceding analysis by controlling explicitly for previous earnings. There was, however, a potentially serious problem of interpretation: the data on prior earnings were obtained directly from patients in the baseline interviews, and the accuracy with which patients recalled and reported their earnings for the previous twelve months is questionable. As a result, it is not clear whether more confidence or less should be placed in the regression results than in the tabulations in tables 6–4 and 6–8.

Effects of Treatment Techniques on Clinical Rating. Table 6–6 reported the differences between E and C patients derived from interviewers' judgments about clinical symptoms. Now we examine the relative effectiveness of E and C approaches within a regression framework, controlling explicitly for the patients' clinical rating at baseline and looking particularly at interactions of diagnostic type with the treatment technology.

Equation 4 simply regresses a patient's score (on a scale from 0, best, to 7, worst) at the end of twelve months of treatment, on that patient's score at baseline, $SLag$, and on a dummy variable for participation in the E program (1 if E).

$$S = 2.25 + 0.25\ SLag - 0.65\ E/C$$
$$(4.25) \quad (2.02) \quad\quad (1.59)$$
$$R^2 = .05 \quad\quad N = 94 \tag{4}$$

There are no surprises, but the prior judgment that the baseline score should be controlled seems to be supported; one additional point on the baseline score was associated with an additional 0.25 of a point after twelve months, suggesting that patients who were more symptomatic at the beginning of the experiment were likely to remain so but with improvement (at a statistically significant level).

The negative sign on E/C is consistent with the table 6–6 results; participation in the E program is associated with an improvement of nearly two-thirds of a point in the clinical score, although the significance level is not high by conventional standards.

Only 5 percent of the variance in S can be explained by the two variables in equation 4. This rises to 18 percent, however, when diagnostic categories are controlled for; in equation 5, dummy variables have been added for nonschizophrenic psychotic, S, and personality disorder, PD, diagnoses, and interaction terms added for each of those diagnostic groups and participation in the E group program.

$$S = 1.65 + 0.16\ SLag - 0.23\ E/C + 2.05\ S$$
$$(2.46) \quad (1.25) \quad\quad (0.36) \quad\quad (3.23)$$
$$+ 0.57\ PD - 1.03\ S*E - 0.17\ PD*E$$
$$(0.86) \quad\quad (1.15) \quad\quad (0.17)$$
$$R^2 = .18 \tag{5}$$

(Complete data on the variables used in equations 4 and 5 were available for only 94 of the total of 130 patients. We are aware of no reason to expect selection bias.)

Using the clinical rating score as the dependent variable, by contrast with earnings, it was found that participation in the E program is associated with somewhat more favorable effects (fewer symptoms) for the PD group (0.17 points on the 7.00 point scale) and considerably more favorable effects for the schizophrenic group (1.03 points), although neither is statistically significant. A comparison of equations 4 and 5, however, shows that the E group schizophrenic patients benefited nearly twice as much, in clinical rating terms (0.23 + 1.03 = 1.26—see equation 5), as the average of all E group patients (0.65 in equation 4); on the other hand, E group patients with personality disorders gained only 0.23 + 0.17 = 0.40 points on the clinical rating.

Conclusion

The specific goal of this chapter is to report the methodology and findings of a benefit-cost analysis of a controlled experiment in the treatment of the mentally ill. In the debate over national health insurance, scant attention has been given to mental illness and even less to the choice among alternative types of delivery systems. The research reported here supports the hypothesis that hospitalization of the mentally ill is, except for emergency situations, less effective than community-based treatment of approximately equal cost.

These empirical findings should be interpreted, however, with caution. The experiment was conducted in one geographic area (Dane County, Wisconsin) during one time interval (October 1972 to March 1976) with each subject participating for only a fourteen-month period. The economic, social, and political environment during that time and in that area could have influenced the experimental findings in important but poorly understood ways. The same experiment operated in a different environment (for example, one with a higher or lower unemployment rate or a larger or smaller city) might have produced substantially different outcomes.

A broader goal of this chapter is to show how any benefit-cost analysis—not simply one in the mental health area—can provide seriously misleading, if not incorrect, results if the range of costs and benefits are not viewed comprehensively and if forms of costs and benefits that are not easily measured in monetary terms are omitted. Empirically, we have found confirmation of the hypothesis that the forms taken by the social costs of alternative programs can be so different that it is easy to mistake a change in the form of costs for a change in their level.

Finally, this chapter has underscored the importance and feasibility, for any benefit-cost analysis, of encompassing all variables deemed relevant, whether or not monetary valuation of them is carried out. Presentation of outcomes in quantitative but nonmonetary terms can be useful, as the analysis presented here has shown.

Moreover, the explicit presentation of even those relevant variables for which no quantitative measures at all can be developed is a desirable part of what the economist can do to inform public policy decisions. Although benefit-cost analysis does not provide a substitute for judgment, it does provide an aid in using judgment.

Notes

1. A helpful textbook is Ezra J. Mishan, *Cost-Benefit Analysis* (New York: Praeger, 1976). Examples of benefit-cost analyses are M. E. Beesley and C. D. Foster, "The Victoria Subway Line: Social Benefit and Finances," *Journal of the Royal Statistical Society* (January 1965), pp. 67–88; Walter Garms, "A Benefit-Cost Analysis of the Upward Bound Program," *Journal of Human Resources*, Spring 1971, pp. 206–220; and Burton Weisbrod, "Costs and Benefits of Medical Research: A Case Study of Poliomyelitis," *The Journal of Political Economy*, vol. 79 (1971), pp. 527–544. For a recent collection of such evaluations, see Robert H. Haveman and Julius Margolis, *Public Policy and Expenditure Analysis* (Chicago: Rand-McNally, 1977). A useful though somewhat dated survey is Alan Prest and Ralph Turvey, "Cost-Benefit Analysis, A Survey," *Economic Journal*, 1965, 685–705. For a theoretic discussion, see Robin Boadway, "The Welfare Foundations of Cost-Benefit Analysis," *Economic Journal* (December 1974), 926–939.

2. On "social experiments," see Alice M. Rivlin, *Systematic Thinking for Social Action* (Washington, D.C.: Brookings Institution, 1971), and Robert Haveman and Harold Watts, "Social Experimentation as Policy Research: A Review of Negative Income Tax Experiments," in Victor Halberstadt and Anthony Culyer, eds., *Public Economics and Human Resources* (Paris: Editions Cajas, 1977); also Glenn V. Glass, ed., *Evaluation Studies Review Annual* (Beverly Hills, California: Sage Publications, 1976).

3. For example, Charles Cipolla, *Public Health and the Medical Professions in the Renaissance* (Cambridge: Cambridge University Press, 1976), p. 57: "Ever since the dawn of civilization, consciously or unconsciously man has always speculated about costs and benefits. Today we use technical jargon and we can turn to impressive statistical information, yet even for contemporary affairs it is almost impossible to reach objective conclusions about costs and benefits when it is a question of health and environment. The fact of the matter is that it is impossible to quantify certain intangibles and a number of value judgments are by necessity subjective and arbitrary." For other critical appraisals, see Arthur Maass, "Benefit-Cost Analysis: Its Relevance to Public Investment Decisions," *Quarterly Journal of Economics*, May 1966, pp. 208–215, and Richard Titmuss, *The Gift Relationship: From Human Blood to Social Policy* (London: George Allen and Unwin Ltd., 1970).

4. Much of the theoretic welfare economics literature on compensation conceives of socially costless, lump-sum, nondistorting taxes and transfers.

More recent work examines the effects of compensation arrangements where distortions are likely. For example, see Joseph Cordes and Burton Weisbrod, "Governmental Behavior in Response to Compensation Requirements," *Journal of Public Economics*, vol. 11 (1979), pp. 47–58.

5. For example, a program to reduce accidents in a subway by reducing the speed of trains might appear to be highly beneficial until it is recognized that the above-ground accident rate rose as subway riders shifted to private autos. Total accident costs could even have increased as the form of cost shifted from subway accidents to road accidents.

6. Other perspectives, such as that of a governmental budget administrator who might be interested simply in cash flows, would produce a different benefit-cost analysis.

7. Indeed, these external effects and interdependent utility functions presumably go far to explain the major role played by the government sector in the treatment of the mentally ill.

8. Benefit-cost analysis in many program areas (nursing homes and securities regulation are two others) must go beyond a narrow criterion of direct beneficiaries' willingness to pay, either because the direct beneficiaries are badly informed and unable to evaluate their benefits and costs, or because external effects are sizable. In either event, benefits to the persons directly involved—as they perceive them—will be erroneous measures of social benefits.

9. A recent book that surveys the literature on valuation of human life is Michael Jones-Lee, *The Value of Life: An Economic Analysis* (Chicago: University of Chicago Press, 1976), especially chapter 2.

10. Virtually all the mental patient's needs are provided within the hospital; the longer the period of hospitalization, the more difficult it is for the patient, once discharged, to cope with the ordinary problems of daily living in the outside world. Outside the hospital the individual's sources of guidance and support are usually sharply reduced. As a result, any new life crisis is likely to find the patient again seeking the shelter of hospital confinement.

11. Two researchers at the Mendota State Hospital—now Mendota Mental Health Institute (MMHI)—Dr. Leonard I. Stein and Dr. Mary Ann Test, developed the treatment program that they felt would avoid this cycle of discharge and rehospitalization. Subsequently, they designed a controlled experiment to test the new treatment model. Dr. Stein, then director of research at MMHI, is now professor of psychiatry, University of Wisconsin-Madison. Dr. Test, a psychologist and former associate director of research at MMHI, is now assistant professor of social work, University of Wisconsin-Madison. For a discussion of the experimental design and treatment approach, see Leonard Stein and Mary Ann Test, "Alternative to Mental Hospital Treatment: I. Conceptual Model, Treatment Program and Clinical Evaluation," *The Archives of General Psychiatry*, April 1980, pp. 392–397.

12. Leonard Stein and Mary Ann Test, "An Alternative to Mental Hospital Treatment: I. Conceptual Model, Treatment Program and Clinical Evaluation," University of Wisconsin-Madison, mimeographed, 1977, pp. 9–10.

13. Data were also collected during a subsequent fourteen-month follow-up phase; this paper, however, deals only with the initial period, for it was only during this interval that different treatment modes were in effect.

14. In a subsequent mental health treatment experiment, some alternative programs were tried (for example, one that reduced the utilization of sheltered workshops), but they were not subjected to an intensive analysis.

15. Providers of services (hospitals, community organizations, etc.) were the major source of data on costs. In some instances, providers gave us figures on average total costs per patient-day or on some other unit of patient contact. They often also gave us information on utilization of their services by patients in the E and C groups, but when they could not or would not provide such information, we fell back on other sources, for example, interviews with patients. In either case, we simply multiplied the average cost figures by the corresponding utilization data to derive the total costs incurred on behalf of the patients in each group. In other instances, service providers gave us data on the total costs incurred in treating or assisting particular patients whose names we provided (without denoting whether the patients were from the E or C group). Property taxes were deducted from the property rental expenditures of the E program, so as to make these costs more comparable to the tax-free, state-owned property occupied by MMHI. We might have chosen, instead, to impute a cost to the MMHI and to estimate the marginal cost of the unpriced public services consumed by both the E and C programs rather than to use property tax payments, actual or imputed. But the additional difficulty of these alternatives and their necessarily conjectural nature supported the use of our alternative. By deducting property tax payments for the E program center and by making no addition to the MMHI cost figure to account for the marginal costs of public services, we have understated the real costs of both the E and C programs; this omission would not bias our finding, however, if the levels of utilization for unpriced public services are similar for the two programs.

16. The E program, unlike the hospital-based C program, started with a patient population of zero; the patient population grew at the rate of 2 to 3 persons per month, reaching a peak of some thirty patients and subsequently declining to zero. (Each patient was in the program for fourteen months, but the entire experiment lasted some three years.) During nearly half of the study the E program had a great deal of slack capacity in the form of underutilized staff time, buildings, and equipment. This over-capacity (resulting from staff indivisibility) led to higher average costs than would have been the case in a steady state. (It also led, however, to more staff time per patient, and thus, perhaps, to higher quality care.)

17. In the judgment of the E program clinical staff, full capacity utiliza-

tion was never reached; thus, our procedure may still overstate long-run equilibrium costs for the E program. By the same token, however, the hospital facility at MMHI, used for the C program, was also operating below capacity—although it operated at essentially a constant level over the study period, by contrast with the variable capacity utilization of the E program.

18. To be sure, it is not likely that all law enforcement costs for each group are attributable to—and hence are costs of—mental illness, but it seems reasonable to attribute differences between the groups to differences in treatment outcomes.

19. Information obtained from the family burden interview is limited in two major respects. The size of the sample is small—49 out of 130—and the follow-up period—four months—is short relative to that of the whole study. (Budgetary constraints and concern about the burden imposed by the interviews themselves limited the number of follow-up interviews.)

20. Because participation in the E treatment program was limited to fourteen months, following which treatment reverted to the conventional C type treatment, family members presumably did not adjust the size of their residence to the temporary absence of the patient. If the E program were made permanent, however, such adjustments would occur, and with them would come reduced housing cost burdens on family members. Thus, in the long run any higher level of maintenance costs for the E program would be at least partially offset by lower family burden costs.

21. To further complicate the matter, some of the real maintenance costs incurred by E group members were probably financed by those patients themselves out of the higher level of their earnings (a variable discussed below in connection with the analysis of benefits). It is social costs, not expenditures per se, that we seek to measure. Direct measurement of the social costs of maintenance was not feasible, however, and so we proxied them by expenditures but were unable to obtain reliable data on patient expenditures, if any, out of their own income.

22. The latter may be interpreted as a reflection of interdependent utility functions, with the health state of the (mentally) ill entering the utility functions of the non-ill, or it may be interpreted as a Rawlsian-type concern by the non-ill about the possibility that they too may someday become ill and in need of outside assistance. Either way, improved mental health per se is a benefit to both patients and others.

23. With respect to patients' reservation wage, it may be useful to consider possible changes over time. Early in the experiment, the E group patients were, to some extent, pressured into working; as a result of this work being involuntary, any increase in the patients' earnings overstates the increase in their real income, given the nature of their utility functions at the time. While the increased earnings (productivity) would constitute a gross benefit from the particular treatment program, the disutility of work would constitute a gross cost. Later in the experiment, however, when patients' utility functions changed in response to therapy, their

attitudes toward work appeared to change; working became more voluntary. During this period the disutility of work became less than the earnings, and, indeed, the disutility might even be negative—as would be the case if the patients got great satisfaction from being able to do socially approved work. The shorter the duration of the early period, the more reasonable the treatment of earnings as a measure of net benefits, for it is during the later period that the assumption of low, or zero, reservation wage is more plausible. (This point grew out of a stimulating conversation with Carl Dahlman.)

24. Workshop clients also require fairly intensive supervision; the cost of this supervision is included in secondary treatment costs.

25. On the choice of a discount rate, see William Baumol, "On the Social Rate of Discount," *American Economic Review*, September 1968, pp. 788–802, and United States Congress, Joint Economic Committee, *Economic Analysis of Public Investment Decisions: Interest Rate Policy and Discounting Analysis* (Washington, D.C., 1968).

26. Jones-Lee, *The Value of Life.*

27. Controlled social experiments in other program areas have raised similar questions about the effects of the limited duration of the experiment and especially about whether behavioral effects (for example, on labor supply) would differ if a program were permanent. See, for example, Charles Metcalf, "Making Inferences from Controlled Income Maintenance Experiments," *American Economic Review*, June 1973, pp. 478–483.

28. See, for example, Arnold C. Harberger, "Three Basic Postulates for Applied Welfare Economics," *Journal of Economic Literature*, September 1971, pp. 785–797.

29. Cordes and Weisbrod, for example, have shown (see note 4) that a government agency required to compensate persons who are harmed as an unintended consequence of its activities may well alter its project selections as a direct result of the distributional (that is, the compensatory) constraint. Thus, distributional equity and allocative efficiency are entwined.

30. In the actual experiment virtually all expenditures of the E program were financed by a federal grant. If the program were introduced, however, in a nonexperimental setting, the state and local governmental roles in financing it would doubtless be sizable.

7

Some Economic Consequences of
Technological Advance
in Medical Care:
The Case of a New Drug

How should a technological change be evaluated? Conceptually, we would like to know whether the present value of its discounted future net benefits is or is not greater than zero. An innovation that imposes increased social costs compared with the counterfactual is not ipso facto inefficient. Neither is an innovation necessarily efficient if it imposes decreased social costs. Both costs and benefits, and their time streams, must be examined.

The technology of medical care encompasses such labor and capital inputs as surgeons and surgical capital, equipment for diagnoses and treatment, and drugs. Given the variety of input combinations available and their expansion over time, the development of expensive new types of inputs, and the widespread use of public and private insurance arrangements that provide incentives for inefficient choice, concern is understandably growing about the rate of increase of medical care expenditures. Whether that concern reflects implicit recognition of allocative inefficiency or of the income redistributions occurring through the governmental tax-transfer system, the political and economic pressures to reduce expenditures for health care are clear.

Written with John Geweke, this paper was prepared for the conference on Drugs and Health: A Reassessment of the Foundations of Public Policy, sponsored by the American Enterprise Institute, November 1979, and published in Robert B. Helms, ed., *Drugs and Health: Economic Issues and Policy Objectives* (Washington, D.C.: American Enterprise Institute, 1981). We thank Donald Roden, of Pracon, Inc., for providing the data, which were made available by the Texas State Medicaid authorities, and Bernd Luedecke for research assistance.

Thus, notwithstanding the economists' social perspective that treats costs and benefits evenhandedly, government policy makers have become increasingly concerned about the effects of innovations on costs alone, especially in the medical care area. It has become a matter of considerable concern that the percentage of gross national product (GNP) devoted to medical care has continued to rise, from 3.5 percent in 1929 to 5.3 percent in 1960 and to 9.1 percent in 1978 (table 7-1). Numerous mechanisms have been discussed and used for the purpose of cost control: deductibles and copayment in health insurance; prepaid group practice (health maintenance organizations—HMOs) and regional hospital planning councils in health care delivery; and prospective reimbursement and second surgical opinions to induce efficiency in the face of health insurance that frequently confronts physicians and patients with zero private marginal costs of care. The Carter administration sought to impose a "cap" on the rate of increase in each hospital's total annual expenditures. Somehow rising total expenditures have come to be regarded as bad irrespective of the (admittedly hard to measure) benefits. In contrast, the percentage of GNP devoted to automobiles has grown for decades without coming to be perceived as a problem, let alone a reflection of allocative inefficiency.

This paper seeks to accomplish two goals: (1) to develop a method for examining the consequences of any new medical care technology and (2) to apply that method to the case of a new drug, cimetidine, used in the treatment of duodenal ulcers. The selection of a drug rather than some other health care input, and of the one specific drug that we consider, was determined by the availability of data. With small modifications, however, the data could be exploited to examine the expenditure consequences of other medical innovations.

The question whether a particular medical input causes medical expenditures to increase or decrease has obvious policy relevance, given the current political emphasis on cost containment. Individual states make decisions, for example, on whether to approve payments for particular drugs and other specific health resources used by Medicaid patients, and the approval process involves consideration of the total effects on expenditures.

Our method, dictated by the twin desires to be conceptually correct and to be operationally relevant, is a simplification of benefit-cost analysis in which benefits from a new technology consist only of reductions in costs and, indeed, reductions in only those costs that are reflected in explicit payments for health resources.

Measuring net benefits by reductions in costs alone results in biased estimates of net benefits, but in general we cannot determine

TABLE 7–1

HEALTH CARE EXPENDITURES IN THE UNITED STATES, 1929–1978

Year	Percentage of GNP	Amount (billions of dollars)
1929	3.5	4
1950	4.5	13
1960	5.3	27
1970	7.6	75
1975	8.6	131
1978	9.1	192

SOURCE: U.S. Department of Commerce, Bureau of the Census, *Statistical Abstract of the United States, 1979*, p. 97.

the direction of bias. If, for example, a new medical technology were to be both more effective in enhancing good health and less costly than the technology it replaced, a focus on costs alone would understate its net social benefits. If the new technology were more effective but also more costly, disregard of the increased effectiveness would lead to the false conclusion that the new technology brought negative net social benefits. If the new technology were both less effective and less costly, measuring its net benefits by the reduction in cost would overstate the net benefits.

Measurement of increased effectiveness is fraught with complexity. If an innovation reduced pain and suffering, we would have a difficult time valuing that benefit. If it led to a strengthening of the body's defense mechanisms so that there were subsequent improvements in health, that would also be difficult to assess; under some circumstances, however, such benefits would appear as reductions in medical care expenditures and thus would be captured by the cost-based approach. What would be overlooked is the value that the affected persons place on their improved health or longevity; reduced expenditures are generally an underestimate of this value.

In the preceding paragraphs we have used the terms "costs" and "expenditures" synonymously. In some contexts this produces misleading conclusions, as in discussions of "inflation" of medical care "costs," which confuse increases in total expenditures on medical care with increases in the prices of a set of inputs of constant quality. To some extent this confusion of costs with expenditures is present in the operational model we set forth here. Ideally, we would measure changes in both benefits and costs. Insofar as we omit some forms of benefits, we are in effect estimating changes in expenditures on a commodity, health status, that is of varying quality, not the cost of producing a commodity of constant quality. This is another way of seeing the possible bias resulting from the systematic omission of those benefits that are not captured by reductions in expenditures. Any observed changes in *expenditures*, in short, do not necessarily imply a change in the *cost* of purchasing a given level of health.

Another variable in the present-value formulation is the "lifetime" of the innovation. Determination of its length is complicated, for that depends on future research and innovation; the length of life of an innovation is a function of when some other medical advance makes that innovation economically obsolete. Though difficult to determine, this variable is likely to be of critical importance. An innovation that is initially more costly than another may be far less costly, as well as more beneficial, in later years; the number of those later years can be crucial to a determination of the present value of the prospective innovation.

The other key variable in the computation of present value is the discount rate. For a long-lived innovation, the value selected for the discount rate can have a great effect on the present value.[1]

Drugs generally used in the treatment of duodenal ulcers include antacids, antidepressants, anticholinergics, and cimetidine. Antacids neutralize the acid in the upper gastrointestinal tract that irritates and prevents the healing of duodenal ulcers. Antidepressants are used to control anxiety, which can exacerbate the symptoms of duodenal ulcers. Anticholinergics block the effect on acid secretion of the stimulant acetylcholine, rather than neutralizing the acid produced as the antacids do. To be effective, however, nearly toxic doses are required; these invariably lead to adverse reactions, such as dry mouth, blurred vision, and retention of urine.

The drug cimetidine was granted a conditional use permit by the Food and Drug Administration (FDA) in September 1977, for use in the treatment of duodenal ulcer and a few other, much rarer disorders of the upper gastrointestinal tract. It is fundamentally different from antacids in that it blocks the production of acid. It differs from the anticholinergics in that it blocks the effect of histamine, which is required for acid secretion. Unlike the anticholinergics, its undesirable side effects appear to be negligible.[2]

Cimetidine is manufactured by Smith Kline & French Laboratories under the trade name Tagamet. The manufacturer claims that the drug promotes rapid ulcer healing and effective symptom relief to a degree unparalleled by clinically acceptable doses of other currently available drugs. This claim seems to be borne out by independent pharmacological studies,[3] but there are no prospective studies on the question of whether or not treatment with cimetidine results in increased recurrence of ulcers when the drug is discontinued. Thus more data are required for an assessment of long-term therapy with cimetidine, but the drug appears to be effective in the short-term treatment of duodenal ulcers.

Although symptoms may subside and healing may occur within the first week or two after treatment with cimetidine begins, that treatment should be continued for four to six weeks. Under the conditions of its approval by the Food and Drug Administration, treatment periods are not to exceed eight weeks. Few side effects greater than those found with placebos have been reported in clinical trials. Sufficient indication for its use is a diagnosis of duodenal ulcers based on a thorough physical examination of the patient and the professional opinion of the examining physician.

Tagamet is generally more expensive in price per dose than other currently available drugs for the treatment of duodenal ulcers: its cost is about three times that of anticholinergics, fifteen times that of sedatives, and thirty times that of antidepressants. One week of therapy using Tagamet costs $8.40, at thirty cents per 300-milligram tablet. It is less clear that the total cost of treatment with Tagamet is greater: it appears that the recommended daily dosage of Tagamet costs about as much as a quantity of antacid that has approximately the same short-term effect.

The outline of this paper is as follows. Having set the stage in this section—that is, having presented a structure for evaluating a new or proposed medical care technology—we turn in the next section to survey previous research that estimates social costs of ulcers and the change in social costs resulting from use of cimetidine. The three following sections present our method for measuring the change in social costs resulting from the new drug, the data base, and our findings.

Social Costs of Duodenal Ulcer Disease

There is a substantial literature devoted to estimating the social costs of various diseases and to ulcers and duodenal ulcers in particular. Much less attention has been given to the effect of changes in medical technology on these costs, the question to which this paper is ultimately addressed. Before describing our approach to this question, we summarize what is known about the social costs of duodenal ulcer and make a preliminary estimate of the likely effect of cimetidine on those costs.

133

Traditionally, social costs associated with any disease have been classified as direct and indirect. Direct costs are the uses in medical care of the disease of resources that have been diverted from other uses. They include hospital care, physicians' services, drug therapy, nursing home expenses, and so on. Indirect costs are those resulting from the loss of current and future productivity due to disability caused by the disease. Measurement of indirect costs is fraught with well-known conceptual problems relating to the valuation of human life and nonmarket activities and to the forecasting of future productivity and interest rates. None of these conventional measures includes the pain, discomfort, and suffering incurred by the patient and his or her family and associates, which are social costs but very difficult to quantify and even more difficult to evaluate.[4]

As we proceed with our examination of the effect of a new medical input on expenditures, note that: (1) a change in expenditures is not equivalent to a change in net costs (costs minus benefits) and (2) the change in expenditures bears no particular relationship to a change in real production costs for the producers or to the profits of the firm or firms that developed or produced the good.

A duodenal ulcer is any tissue death that results in a crater on the mucous membrane of the duodenum, which is the first ten to twelve inches of the small intestine. The immediate physiological cause is unknown. It is a chronic, recurrent disease characterized by sporadic episodes of acute symptoms. The pain is usually not localized; it may occur daily or may be periodic, lasting for seven to ten days followed by periods of no pain, and may be very intense. A commonly used analogy is that gastric acid dripping on an open ulcer is like boiling water being poured onto a burn. Current techniques for diagnosis are expensive, unpleasant for the patient, and time consuming.

In the treatment of duodenal ulcers the patient is "managed" through symptomatic relief by diet control and liberal use of antacids while the ulcer heals itself, usually in six to eight weeks. Although most patients respond well without surgery, recurrence of the disease for those patients is common. Only about 25 percent of patients with newly diagnosed duodenal ulcers eventually require surgery, and only 10 to 25 percent of these experience permanent remission of all symptoms. Even if the treatment seems effective and the symptoms abate, the sporadic and recurrent nature of ulcer pain requires that the patient be monitored over a considerable period to determine whether the ulcer is dormant or has indeed healed.

An important social characteristic of duodenal ulcers is that it seems to be a life-style disease. That is, certain ways of living and kinds of activities may increase its occurrence in the population. (Lung cancer, coronary disease, and obesity are other examples of life-style diseases.) Although psychiatrists no longer believe that the characterization of the "ulcer personality" as hard-driving, ambitious, over-achieving, and competitive is accurate, they have observed that many ulcer patients need to be dependent but fight that need.

A pattern of regular living with few emotional upsets is therefore a vital ingredient in the long-term management of ulcer patients. This pattern may, of course, be very difficult to bring about. Ulcers that refuse to heal may eventually lead to various complications— among them minor or major bleeding. The mortality rate for bleeding from a duodenal ulcer is about 10 percent; for massive bleeding it is 14 to 25 percent.

If such conditions develop, hospitalization of the patient is invariably required and surgery is frequently required. There are other reasons why a provider may hospitalize a patient: a long history of duodenal ulcers that are not responsive to medical management, a home environment unlikely to reinforce compliance with a therapeutic regimen, or a job that makes therapeutic compliance a practical impossibility.

Most social cost estimates have been undertaken for peptic ulcers, which include all ulcer diseases of the digestive system, rather than for duodenal ulcers alone. Robinson Associates have estimated that 68 percent of peptic ulcer social costs should be ascribed to duodenal ulcer; this figure permits some rough inferences about social costs of duodenal ulcer disease from social cost studies of peptic ulcers.[5]

The results of earlier studies have been reviewed and updated by von Haunalter and Chandler.[6] They estimate that, in 1975, 4 million U.S. residents suffered from some form of ulcer disease. There were 6,840 deaths attributed to ulcer in that year, and 77,000 persons were disabled. Their total social cost estimate for 1975 is $2.6 billion. Direct costs account for slightly less than half of this total, but they are increasing more rapidly than indirect costs. The largest cost component is morbidity, divided fairly evenly between those disabled by ulcer and those temporarily absent from work. The reduced productivity of ulcer sufferers who work at a slower pace is not included because it is nearly impossible to measure it.

The only effort that has been made to evaluate the likely affect of the introduction of cimetidine on the social costs attributed to duodenal ulcer was the study by Robinson Associates, which was commissioned by Smith Kline & French Laboratories. In that study, twenty-three of the physicians who conducted clinical trials of cimetidine for the Food and Drug Administration were asked to describe in detail their drug treatment regimens for various types of duodenal ulcer patients with and without cimetidine. They were asked to evaluate both regimens according to the criteria of frequency of repeat episodes, frequency of patients' visits to physicians, likelihood and frequency of hospitalization, likelihood of surgery, frequency of diagnostic X-rays and endoscopies, amount of missed work, and likelihood of death from ulcer complications. These estimates were then combined with information from secondary sources on indirect costs and costs of various forms of treatment to compute cost reductions resulting from the availability of cimetidine for each type of duodenal ulcer patient. The physicians were also asked to estimate a penetration rate for cimetidine—that is, the percentage of each type of patient that would be treated with cimetidine when the drug was being used by most of the physicians in the United States who would eventually do so.

The findings of this study are summarized in table 7–2. At the average estimated penetration rate of 80 percent, a reduction of $645 million, or 29 percent, in health care costs for duodenal ulcer was estimated. The drug cost component was estimated to increase by 40 percent, but decreases were estimated in all other components. The authors of the study claim that because the sample of twenty-three physicians constituted a carefully selected group of experienced respondents offering highly technical information on a subject with which they were more familiar than any other physicians in the United States, a high degree of confidence may be placed in their assessments. The study provides no quantitative assessment of that confidence, however.

Method

The method developed here for measuring the socioeconomic costs and benefits of the introduction of a new drug is general enough to be used in the evaluation of any new drug, although we focus specifically on cimetidine. In the introduction of any new drug, it is all but impossible to evaluate economic and social effects—as distinguished from medical effects—through a controlled experiment. Besides inherent political and ethical problems, the costs of designing and monitoring such an experiment plus the cost of introducing yet another delay in the introduction of new drugs are apt to be prohibitive. For the foreseeable future, inferences about socioeconomic effects must therefore be drawn in nonexperimental settings, often using data bases constructed for other purposes. These problems are paramount in the evaluation of cimetidine, and we believe they are

TABLE 7–2

Costs of Duodenal Ulcers, Computed for 80 Percent Cimetidine Use, 1977

Cost Component	Total National Costs (millions of dollars)		National Costs per Patient (dollars)		Percentage Reduction
	Amount	Reduction	Amount	Reduction	
Direct costs					
Hospital care	474	258	225	123	35
Physicians and related	139	47	66	23	26
Drug therapy	119	−34	57	−16	−40
Nursing home	11	—	5	—	0
Other professional	2	—	1	—	0
Total direct costs	745	271	351	130	27
Indirect costs					
Mortality	201	44	96	21	18
Morbidity	602	329	286	156	35
Absenteeism	307	148	146	70	33
Long-term disability	295	181	140	86	38
Total indirect costs	803	373	381	177	32
Total	1,547	645	732	307	29

SOURCE: Robinson Associates, *Impact of Cimetidine*, pp. 2–3.

likely to be of overriding concern in the introduction of other drugs and medical techniques as well. The method devised here to cope with the problems of nonexperimental design should be applicable in other cases.

A Hypothetical Experiment. To highlight the difficulties of making inferences about socioeconomic effects in nonexperimental settings, imagine that a controlled experiment could be constructed in which duodenal ulcer patients and providers were randomly assigned to three groups: group 1, in which the key treatment variable, cimetidine, was not available; group 2, in which the use of cimetidine was mandatory; and group 3, in which cimetidine was available but its use was not mandatory. Group 1 might be termed the control group, C; groups 2 and 3, the experimental groups, E_1 and E_2. In many controlled experiments in the health area, only groups C and E_1 are compared. This approach can be quite misleading if the most effective therapy is to use the experimental variable (cimetidine in this case) only some of the time. Whether our group E_2 patients would or would not use cimetidine would depend on providers' judgments. Clearly the more interesting experiment is a comparison of groups C and E_2.[7]

The social costs associated with each of the two groups, C and E_2, would be monitored over a period of time. One possible relationship of the social cost paths of the two groups is illustrated in figure 7–1. During the preexperimental period, social costs for the two randomly chosen groups are the same, because of the controlled nature of the experiment. Early in the experimental period, some patients in E_2 would be treated with cimetidine and perhaps other therapies as well. Since cimetidine treatment normally lasts about eight weeks, drug costs per patient for the experimental group might be expected to be higher early in the experimental period. As the experiment proceeds, however, it could be hypothesized that the social costs associated with the E_2 group would be lower than those of the control group. For a chronic disease like duodenal ulcers, complete measurement of social costs might well require an experimental period of many years. The net social cost saving from the introduction of cimetidine would simply be the difference between the area marked B and that marked A in figure 7–1 after appropriate discounting for passage of time.

This hypothetical experiment has two attractive features in common with any well-designed experiment, of which one is always absent in nonexperimental situations and the other is likely to be absent. The first is that the "fairness" of the trial is guaranteed by random assignment of patients and providers. In the actual introduction of any new drug, assignment is made by the actors themselves —primarily providers but, to varying degrees, the patients as well. There are two problems here. First, we have no practical way of knowing whether those providers and patients who use the new technology differ in important ways from those who do not. It could be that as soon as the new drug is approved for conditional use by the FDA, all providers have access to it and are fully aware of how it should be used in conjunction with other treatments; but this case is rather implausible. It might also be that all patients receive the drug just introduced; but this case is also unlikely. If neither of these polar cases prevails, systematic differences between the experimental and control groups are likely to exist. In particular, patients whose social costs are higher may well be proportionately more important in one group than in the other. The obvious bias that this nonproportional representation introduces in measurements of the type illustrated in figure 7–1 is an example of the selectivity bias that can exist whenever

FIGURE 7–1

HYPOTHETICAL COSTS PER PATIENT,
EXPERIMENTAL AND CONTROL GROUPS

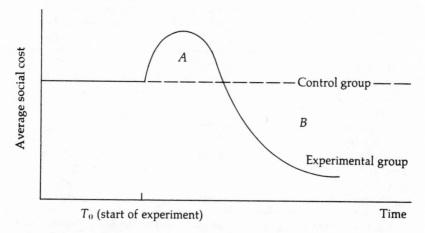

inferences are made in nonexperimental settings under the erroneous assumption of random assignment.

The second attractive feature of our hypothetical experiment is that extensive measures of socioeconomic well-being can be made, provided the control and experimental groups are kept small enough that the costs of measurement are not prohibitive. In nonexperimental situations this is usually not the case, although it could be: intensive measurements of a randomly selected subpopulation could be made, as they are for the general population by the Bureau of the Census and the Bureau of Labor Statistics each month. Most of the existing measures, however, have been made for the entire population. Like the data discussed in the previous section, they have insufficient coverage and detail because they are collected for other purposes.

Making Inferences from Nonexperimental Data. It seems unlikely that either of the two polar cases discussed would prevail in practice, and in the introduction of cimetidine there is some evidence that they did not. The FDA certified effectiveness of the new drug only for duodenal ulcers and some hypersecretory conditions that are rare by comparison. In our sample, however, we were able to associate only about one of every fourteen prescriptions of cimetidine with a diagnosis of duodenal ulcer. Since the providers' behavior and the FDA certification restrictions cannot both reflect optimal use of the drug, the first case is ruled out.[8] In the other polar case, in which

TABLE 7-3

Use of Cimetidine, September 1977–June 1978

	Distribution of Prescriptions (n = 530)	Ratio of Cimetidine-Treated Patients to New Patients Not So Treated[a] (n = 1,206)
September 1977	0.057	0.698
October 1977	0.100	0.946
November 1977	0.098	1.182
December 1977	0.134	1.164
January 1978	0.098	0.839
February 1978	0.160	1.308
March 1978	0.075	0.571
April 1978	0.087	0.719
May 1978	0.094	0.667
June 1978	0.096	0.375

a. A new duodenal ulcer patient is one whose first indication of duodenal ulcer in the period September 1977–June 1978 occurred in the month indicated.
Source: Author.

all duodenal ulcer patients receive cimetidine, the penetration rate should increase toward unity, and the ratio of patients treated with cimetidine to those not treated should increase without bound. Table 7-3 shows, however, that this was decidedly not the case for the Texas Medicaid sample.

The Medicaid data, being nonexperimental, do not permit separate analyses of the E_1 and E_2 groups. We know only that some providers prescribed cimetidine to some patients, and so we have an approximation to group E_2. There is no group E_1, for which cimetidine therapy was mandatory. (It is also notable that we can distinguish between those cimetidine users for whom duodenal ulcers were diagnosed and other users of the drug.)

We identify all duodenal ulcer patients who received cimetidine between September 1, 1977, and June 30, 1978, as the T group, all other patients who received treatment (but not cimetidine) for duodenal ulcer during that period as the F group. We control for selectivity bias within the limitations imposed by the data base. With a sufficiently large sample, we would restrict our attention to patients with indications of an active ulcer diagnosis in the period P, September 1, 1977, to June 30, 1978; a patient is assumed to have an active ulcer problem if any treatment is provided for duodenal ulcer as a primary or secondary diagnosis or if he or she is treated with an antiulcer drug and has a diagnosis of duodenal ulcer during the preceding year. The timing of indicators of socioeconomic cost for each patient is measured from the first indication of an active ulcer within the sample period for those in group F and from the prescription of cimetidine for those in group T. This point of reference is the analogue of the start of a controlled environment and corresponds to the point T_0 in figure 7-1. For group F the point of reference chosen is the first indication of ulcer rather than September 1 because, if the date were chosen, some patients with no active ulcer problem at the reference point would be included in F, whereas all patients in T do have an active ulcer problem at the time cimetidine is prescribed. Presumably there would then be a downward bias in the measurement of social costs for group F relative to group T and an upward bias in the estimated cost-reducing effects of cimetidine.

Samples F and T are subdivided to control for all measured factors that might affect real treatment costs. The divisions are made conditional on two groups of variables.

The variables in the first group are demographic: the sex, race, and age of each patient are known, and our sample may be divided on the basis of these variables. There is an obvious and large potential for selectivity bias if demographic factors are ignored. (As we shall see, even if all demographic groups were identical with respect to the relevant medical factors and were proportioned in the same way between F and T, there would still be reason to separate them in assessing social medical care costs.)

The second group of variables consists of those associated with the "severity" of a given disease. Under nonexperimental circumstances, we can never adequately measure all those factors that would be controlled implicitly in a randomized experiment. Even in the experiment contemplated above, providers may (even subconsciously) take into account unmeasured or unmeasurable dimensions of a patient's health in deciding whether or not to prescribe cimetidine. There is no way to account for nonrandom factors that affect assignment to groups F and T but are uncorrelated with measured variables. The best that one can do is to account adequately for the variables that are measured.

In the present study, there are available four specific variables that, it is reasonable to assume, are associated with potentially nonrandom assignment and that are related to social costs. All relate to a specified period before the reference point, which we will call the presample period. They are (1) the number of indications of sickness; (2) expenditures on health care; (3) days hospitalized; and (4) indications of other disease. Each may be positively correlated with medical care costs over the presample period and over the sample period, whether cimetidine was prescribed or not. Failure to account for these variables could introduce a potentially very large source of selectivity bias: one has only to imagine polar situations in which providers prescribe cimetidine only to patients at death's door or, alternatively, cimetidine is given only to those who are relatively healthy or are on no other medication and consequently are unlikely to suffer complications.

In principle, selectivity bias would be minimized by controlling for each of these factors when evaluating treatment costs, using a very fine categorization, but this can lead to more cells than observations. We tested for the existence of selectivity bias for each of seven dimensions (sex, race, age, indications of sickness, expenditures on health care, days of hospitalization, and indications of other disease) by testing the hypothesis that the proportion receiving cimetidine is unaffected by variations in that dimension in the presample period. We control for selectivity bias by subdividing the sample only in those cases where such bias appeared to be substantively and statistically significant. Once this initial subdivision was made, we tested for selectivity bias within each subsample and made further subdivisions only where there was evidence within a subsample of selectivity bias on another dimension. The subsamples so selected are the populations within which treatment costs associated with the new technology, incorporating cimetidine, and the old are compared.

Measurement of Social Cost Variables. Having subdivided our sample in this way, we have now approximated the conditions of controlled experiments undertaken on each of a number of groups of patients. The proportion of patients receiving cimetidine is in general not the same in each subsample; this, indeed, necessitated the subdivision of the original sample to reduce selectivity bias. Within each group, we monitor indicators of social cost in the fashion anticipated in figure 7–1, the subdivisions and testing procedures outlined above providing some assurance that the paths of measurable treatment cost variables in the presample period are about the same for the F and T groups in each subsample, as they would be expected to be in a randomized experimental design.

At this point, further division of the sample may be desirable. Tests for selectivity bias, for example, may indicate no need to dissociate young males from older females, but it is quite conceivable that the two groups might respond very differently to cimetidine and other treatments in the sample period. Since the socioeconomic implications of the ability to control a chronic disease indefinitely are very different for the two groups, they would be analyzed separately. In the interests of manageability, however, we treat groups separately only if separation is necessary to reduce (and, we hope, eliminate) selection bias or if groups with different socioeconomic characteristics behave in the sample period in ways that are statistically significantly different.

For each group, we estimate the mean and standard deviation of paths of the form shown in figure 7–1. For continuous variables like health care expenditures, the quantity estimated is the expected value for a patient in the group at a particular time in relation to the reference point. For categorical variables like "no days hospitalized," the estimated quantity is a probability. From the nature of our sample, it is obvious that the position of the path is estimated with less accuracy as one moves to the right of the reference point, especially for group T, because the sample becomes thinner. Means and probabilities for the whole ten-month sample period are also estimated. By weighting the numerical importance of each group treated separately, we arrive at estimates of magnitudes associated with treatment costs.

Data Base

All the data used in this study are taken from Medicaid claims in Texas for the period September 1976 through June 1978. The data were collected originally for accounting purposes and were made available to us by Pracon, an independent consulting firm of Fairfax, Virginia. Pracon and SysteMetrics, of Santa Barbara, California, converted the data from their original form to a form more suitable for studying the health care experience of individual patients.

The basic organizational unit from which our files were constructed is a claim—a bill submitted to the state of Texas for a medical service or drug. When a claim had been amended after its original submission, the amended claim was used. Associated with each claim are a patient identification number; an identification number for the provider (for example, a physician or pharmacy); a primary and sometimes a secondary diagnosis if the claim is for hospital, physician, or nursing home services; the date of the claim; the date on which the service was rendered; the nature of the service performed by the physician (for example, surgery or consultation); the length of stay in a hospital or nursing home; the amount of a drug provided; and the dollar amount of the claim. Demographic information—sex, race, and age—about each patient is provided, as is detailed information about the provider: for example, the specialty of physicians and whether a hospital is profit, nonprofit, or a unit of an institution.

Perhaps the most attractive feature of this data base is the detailed medical information about the period in which health care costs are incurred as well as the time at which they are billed. Together with patient identification numbers, this information makes possible a detailed reconstruction of that portion of a patient's health care that was paid for by the state. Although we believe that this data set constitutes the best nonexperimental evidence yet assembled for the evaluation of innovations in medical technology, it is not without its shortcomings. Those that follow are most important in limiting the kinds of questions that can be addressed or in evaluating the results presented here:

- The only aspects of patients' experiences that are known to us are those that entail a claim. In particular, there is no direct information on morbidity outside institutions. At most, we can make rough guesses about the implications for work experience of days hospitalized and of various diagnoses and drug prescriptions.

- Only those direct costs billable to the state Medicaid system are known; there is no way of knowing the nature or magnitude of other health care costs. For patients over sixty-five the problem is significant, because many of their health care costs are paid by Medicare. For those under sixty-five Medicaid generally pays all health care bills for eligible recipients.

- In the case of duodenal ulcer, there is little information available about the severity of the illness. Diagnoses are recorded using the International Classification of Diseases, which provides eight gradations of severity for duodenal ulcer, but most providers use the code for a ninth classification in which severity is unspecified. Hence we have little information about a potentially important source of selectivity bias.

- For drug claims, no diagnosis is indicated. Hence it is not possible to get reliable information on the drug therapy component of direct costs for cimetidine-based and non-cimetidine-based treatments.

- Deaths are not recorded in our data set. If a higher proportion of patients in one group died, we would observe lower expenditures on medical care for that group.

It should also be noted that our data are limited to Medicaid patients. We do not believe that they constitute a biased sample of the entire duodenal ulcer population in relation to the expenditure effects of cimetidine, but we cannot be certain.

From the original file of about 12 million claims, the sample S was constructed as described in the previous section. This sample is restricted to those who were eligible for the Medicaid program during the entire period September 1976 through June 1978. Sample T is composed of those in S with a diagnosis of duodenal ulcer on some claim from September 1976 through June 1978 who also had a claim for cimetidine from September 1977 through June 1978. Sample F is composed of those in S with a diagnosis of duodenal ulcer on some claim from September 1976 through June 1978 who had either a claim with a duodenal ulcer diagnosis or a claim for an ulcer prescription— but not cimetidine—during that period. For the latter group, "ulcer prescription" is defined by the National Drug Commission codes, and base dating begins with the first such claim or prescription between September 1977 and June 1978. There are 1,206 persons in sample S, of whom 530 are in sample T.

Findings

In this section we report our estimates of the changes in certain public expenditures and other measures of costs that may be ascribed to the introduction of the new medical technology incorporating cimetidine. After briefly discussing selectivity biases evident in the data, we treat total health care expenditures, expenditures on hospitals and physicians for duodenal ulcer, and days of hospitalization. All three measures can be disaggregated in various ways, but a careful discussion at this level of detail is beyond the scope of this paper.

By any number of measures, it appears that the new drug has been administered to patients who exhibited more illness in the preceding twelve months than did those patients treated with older therapies (table 7–4). Patients treated with cimetidine were hospitalized almost 50 percent more days than those who were not in the preceding twelve months—7.46 days compared with 5.14—and their total health care expenditures for this period were significantly higher, $1,506 compared with $1,293.

A close examination of monthly expenditure and hospitalization records reveals that much of the difference between the two groups' presample histories occurs in the month immediately preceding the base date. This difference may be accounted for by the environment in which cimetidine is prescribed and by our definition of the base date. For patients who receive cimetidine, any immediately preceding duodenal ulcer therapy is by definition in the presample period; for patients who do not receive cimetidine, our sample is so constructed that there can be no duodenal ulcer therapy in the immediately

TABLE 7-4
Tests for Selectivity Bias

Variable	Sample T (N = 676) Mean	Standard deviation	Sample F (N = 530) Mean	Standard deviation	t-value
Days hospitalized, −12/−1	7.46	111.00	5.14	9.57	−3.84***
Total expenditures, −12/−1 (dollars)	1,506.0	2,224.0	1,293.0	1,945.0	−1.72*
Drugs	125.0	110.0	111.0	109.0	−2.18**
Outpatient	74.8	181.0	44.9	118.0	−3.28***
Hospital	674.0	1,314.0	499.0	1,096.0	−2.45**
Physicians	278.0	1,476.0	231.0	370.0	−1.88*
Physician and hospital expenditures with diagnosis of duodenal ulcer, −12/−1	117.0	376.0	60.5	219.0	−3.07
Days hospitalized, −12/−2	5.33	9.57	4.44	8.51	−1.69*
Total expenditures, −12/−2 (dollars)	1,280.0	2,014.0	1,138.0	1,826.0	−1.26
Drugs	113.0	102.0	100.0	100.0	−2.20**
Outpatient	65.6	162.0	38.2	100.0	−3.41***
Hospital	542.0	1,177.0	434.0	1,005.0	−1.68*
Physicians	241.0	431.0	203.0	338.0	−1.63
Physician and hospital expenditures with diagnosis of duodenal ulcer, −12/−2 (dollars)	61.5	316.0	54.7	212.0	−0.42

* Significant at 10 percent level. ** Significant at 5 percent level. *** Significant at 1 percent level.
SOURCE: Author.

preceding month—only therapy for other diagnoses—unless the treatment occurred during September 1977. There is, however, a problem of selectivity bias independent of how the first presample month should be treated. For the first eleven months of the presample period, cimetidine patients still exhibited greater health problems in the seven dimensions exhibited in table 7-4, although the differences are smaller than when the first presample month is included and are

146

significantly different at the 10 percent level in only four instances.

Examination of demographic variables turned up no significant differences between the two groups. Expenditures associated with the treatment of duodenal ulcer in the first eleven months of the presample period averaged only a few dollars per month per patient and were not significantly different for the T and F samples. Both health care expenditures and days of hospitalization in the presample period affected the probability that a given patient would be treated with cimetidine. Because of the size of the sample, stratification was attempted only on total health care expenditures in the first eleven months of the presample period.

Because of the special behavior of the history of health care in the first presample month in the T and F samples, we have treated this month in two different ways in reporting our results. In essence, the question is whether treatment received immediately before a cimetidine prescription is an integral part of the new technology that incorporates cimetidine. If it is, then expenditures incurred in the first presample month should be associated with cimetidine, and comparing expenditures for the T and F samples beginning with the base date would lead to a downward bias in the expenditure estimate for the T sample. In all likelihood, expenditures in the first month of the presample are part of the new technology for some patients treated with cimetidine (for example, those whose newly diagnosed ulcer was confirmed by an endoscopy) but are not for others (for example, those for whom the new technology was used after other methods failed). In the estimates reported below, we compare samples T and F for three months, -1 through $+2$; for two months -1 and $+1$; and for the single month $+1$. The cost of the treatment of therapy incorporating cimetidine in relation to that not incorporating cimetidine is probably overstated for the first two groups of months and understated for the last.

In tables 7–5, 7–6, and 7–7 we report mean total health care expenditures, expenditures for hospitals and physicians for persons with a diagnosis of duodenal ulcer, and days of hospitalization for several interesting subperiods of the presample and postsample periods. In all cases we eliminated from the sample patients over sixty-five because expenditure records for patients eligible for Medicare are incomplete. In each table the sample has been stratified by total health care expenditures in the first eleven months of the presample period: less than $300 (group A), $300 to $1,000 (group B), and more than $1,000 (group C). Overall means have also been computed, by weighting groups A, B, and C by their proportionate representation in the entire sample of patients under sixty-five.

TABLE 7-5
HEALTH CARE EXPENDITURES

Control Group[a]	Month	T Sample			F Sample			t-value
		N	Mean ($)	Standard deviation ($)	N	Mean ($)	Standard deviation ($)	
A	−12/ −2	149	113	93.5	206	95.3	90.1	−1.83*
	−1/ +1	149	504	781	206	745	1,460	2.00**
	+1	149	325	658	206	663	1,404	3.01***
	−1/ +2	139	569	781	190	835	1,432	2.15**
	+2/ +4	116	316	580	151	313	772	−0.02
	+5/ +7	57	264	570	81	154	337	−1.30
	+8/+10	10	79.6	68.7	31	202	434	1.51
B	−12/ −2	97	543	184	127	594	196	1.99**
	−1/ +1	97	449	709	127	481	866	0.31
	+1	97	305	593	127	359	711	0.61
	−1/ +2	92	587	770	119	576	889	−0.09
	+2/ +4	65	335	540	95	383	719	0.48
	+5/ +7	37	205	383	64	459	790	2.16**

C	+8/ +10	16	150	215	18	511	806	1.82*
	−12/ −2	132	3,432	2,581	149	2,951	2,265	−1.65
	−1/ +1	132	900	1,204	149	736	938	−1.25
	+1	132	511	913	149	423	678	−0.90
	−1/ +2	125	1,114	1,316	140	1,068	1,292	0.78
	+2/ +4	101	878	1,272	117	863	1,170	−0.08
	+5/ +7	44	694	1,109	76	598	832	−0.49
	+8/+10	10	929	1,088	33	691	1,432	−0.55
Overall	−12/ −2	378	1,310	1,480	482	1,159	1,300	−1.57
	−1/ 11	378	619	926	482	673	1,167	0.76
	+1	378	381	737	482	506	1,047	2.05**
	−1/ +2	356	752	986	449	844	1,264	1.16
	+2/ +4	282	505	862	363	511	910	0.09
	+5/ +7	138	389	758	189	378	660	−0.14
	+8/+10	36	376	544	82	442	957	0.47

NOTE: The overall means are computed by weighting groups A, B, and C by their proportions in the population: 0.413, 0.260, and 0.327, respectively.

* Significant at 10 percent level.

** Significant at 5 percent level.

*** Significant at 1 percent level.

a. Patients under sixty-five with less than $300 total health care expenditures in months −12/−2 of the presample period constitute group A; $300 to $1,000, group B; over $1,000, group C.

SOURCE: Author.

TABLE 7-6

EXPENDITURES FOR HOSPITALS AND PHYSICIANS FOR DUODENAL ULCERS

Control Group [a]	Month	T Sample			F Sample			t-value
		N	Mean ($)	Standard deviation ($)	N	Mean ($)	Standard deviation ($)	
A	−12/ −2	149	4.39	22.6	206	3.55	14.9	− 0.39
	−1/ +1	149	173	514	206	447	1,257	2.81***
	+1	149	108	445	206	438	1,258	3.47***
	−1/ +2	139	196	533	190	439	1,261	2.37**
	+2/ +4	116	51.2	170	151	36.3	217	−0.62
	+5/ +7	57	95.2	357	81	7.91	45.1	−1.83*
	+8/+10	10	0	0	31	23.6	116	1.12
B	−12/ −2	97	47.7	127	127	61.7	142	0.77
	−1/ +1	97	124	293	127	146	435	0.43
	+1	97	98.0	271	127	144	435	0.98
	−1/ +2	92	139	304	119	136	364	−0.06
	+2/ +4	65	51.5	207	95	23.2	104	−1.01
	+5/ +7	37	4.93	22.6	64	14.5	79.0	0.90
	+8/+10	16	.849	3.39	18	25.8	109	0.96

C							
−12/ −2	132	166	603	149	143	409	−0.35
−1/ +1	132	167	918	149	197	505	0.55
+1	132	97.4	339	149	187	498	1.79*
−1/ +2	125	167	386	140	211	517	0.78
+2/ +4	101	60.2	228	117	42.2	241	−0.56
+5/ +7	44	29.2	170	76	63.6	364	0.70
+8/ +10	10	0	0	33	8.90	35.6	1.43
Overall							
−12/ −2	378	68.5	351	482	64.3	245	−0.20
−1/ +1	378	158	638	482	287	886	2.48**
+1	378	102	372	482	279	885	3.97***
−1/ +2	356	171	436	449	286	882	2.42**
+2/ +4	282	54.2	200	363	34.8	203	−1.21
+5/ +7	138	50.2	244	189	27.8	214	−0.86
+8/ +10	36	.221	1.73	82	19.4	95.1	1.82*

NOTE: The overall means are computed by weighting groups A, B, and C by their proportions in the population: 0.413, 0.260, and 0.327, respectively.

* Significant at 10 percent level.
** Significant at 5 percent level.
*** Significant at 1 percent level.

a. Patients under sixty-five with less than $300 total health care expenditures in months −12/ −2 of the presample period constitute group A; $300 to $1,000, group B; over $1,000, group C.

SOURCE: Author.

TABLE 7-7
Days of Hospitalization

Control Group[a]	Month	T Sample			F Sample			t-value
		n	Mean	Standard deviation	n	Mean	Standard deviation	
A	−12/ −2	149	0.19	0.12	216	0.14	1.06	−0.34
	−1/ +1	149	2.41	3.99	206	4.02	6.18	2.97***
	+1	149	1.49	3.39	206	3.68	5.48	4.36***
	−1/ +2	139	2.51	3.74	190	4.50	6.61	3.45***
	+2/ +4	116	1.18	2.92	151	1.31	3.54	0.32
	+5/ +7	57	1.22	3.37	81	.703	2.15	−1.03
	+8/+10	10	0	0.00	31	.806	2.18	2.06**
B	−12/ −2	97	2.04	5.38	127	2.21	2.75	0.28
	−1/ +1	97	2.23	4.02	127	2.64	5.06	0.67
	+1	97	1.36	3.26	127	2.00	4.21	1.28
	−1/ +2	92	2.86	4.32	119	3.48	6.86	0.79
	+2/ +4	65	2.35	6.06	95	2.30	6.13	−0.04
	+5/ +7	37	0.70	2.41	64	1.89	3.97	1.86*
	+8/+10	16	0	0	18	3.00	7.12	1.78*

C	−12/ −2	132	14.4	12.1	149	13.2	11.9	−0.81
	−1/ +1	132	4.71	6.33	149	3.47	5.99	−1.68*
	+1	132	2.59	4.74	149	2.10	4.12	−0.92
	−1/ +2	125	5.69	6.79	140	4.65	7.05	−1.22
	+2/ +4	101	3.82	6.54	117	3.25	6.03	−0.65
	+5/ +7	44	3.77	7.50	76	1.73	3.34	−1.70*
	+8/ +10	10	3.90	6.75	33	1.48	3.34	−1.09
Overall	−12/ −2	378	5.32	7.44	482	4.95	6.98	−0.74
	−1/ +1	378	3.11	4.89	482	3.48	5.85	1.01
	+1	378	1.82	3.85	482	2.73	4.75	3.10***
	−1/ +2	356	3.64	5.07	449	4.28	6.82	1.53
	+2/ +4	282	2.35	5.20	363	2.20	5.18	−0.05
	+5/ +7	138	1.92	4.96	189	1.35	3.11	−1.19
	+8/ +10	36	1.28	3.86	82	1.60	4.34	0.40

NOTE: The overall means are computed by weighting groups A, B, and C by their proportions in the population: 0.413, 0.260, and 0.327, respectively.

* Significant at 10 percent level.
** Significant at 5 percent level.
*** Significant at 1 percent level.

a. Patients under sixty-five with less than $300 total health care expenditures in months −12/−2 of the presample period constitute group A; $300 to $1,000, group B; over $1,000, group C.

SOURCE: Author.

It is perhaps worth emphasizing that the overall means for T and F are not the simple means. Because the simple means would reflect the higher proportion of patients in sample T who had high presample health care expenditures, the simple means do not control for the selection bias inherent in the data. Patients with high (and intermediate and low) presample health care expenditures are of equal importance in the overall means for samples T and F.

All groups and samples show high mean expenditures and mean days of hospitalization immediately after the base date, followed by a decrease that is sometimes sharp but does not usually return to presample levels (see, for example, figures 7–2 to 7–5, for expenditures). In the first month or two of the sample period, almost all patients have higher expenditures than in the presample period; but in the later months of the sample period, a few patients have high expenditures and many (in some instances, most) have no expenditures at all in a given month, as reflected in standard deviations greater than the mean for all but one entry for the months $+2/+4$, $+5/+7$, and $+8/+10$ in tables 7–5 and 7–6. The data on which table 7–6 is based are less reliable than those for tables 7–5 and 7–7, because diagnostic information is often not reported by hospitals and physicians.

Systematic and significant differences emerge only early in the sample period and only for group A, which had the lowest presample health care expenditures. For the patients who received cimetidine, overall health care expenditures (table 7–5) were 32 percent lower in months $-1/+2$ (which we have argued provides a lower bound on relative costs) and 51 percent in month $+1$ (the upper bound). Expenditures for hospitals and physicians with an associated diagnosis of duodenal ulcer (table 7–6) were 55 percent lower in months $-1/+2$ and 75 percent lower in month $+1$, and mean days of hospitalization (table 7–7) were 44 percent lower in months $-1/+2$ and 60 percent lower in month $+1$. In the later months of the sample period, differences in expenditures and in hospitalization for the two samples are for the most part statistically insignificant. These differences are small arithmetically as well and do not appear to result from the fact that the sample becomes smaller as we move further beyond the base date.

For the two groups with higher health care expenditures in the presample period, groups B and C, differences between the T and F samples during the sample period are mostly statistically insignificant. Perhaps the technology that incorporates cimetidine does not, in fact, reduce health care costs for patients with more severe health problems. The proportionate reduction in total health care expenditures would be less, however, to the extent that "more severe health problems"

FIGURE 7–2

AVERAGE TOTAL HEALTH CARE EXPENDITURES,
PERSONS UNDER SIXTY-FIVE,
$0–300 EXPENDITURES IN PRESAMPLE YEAR

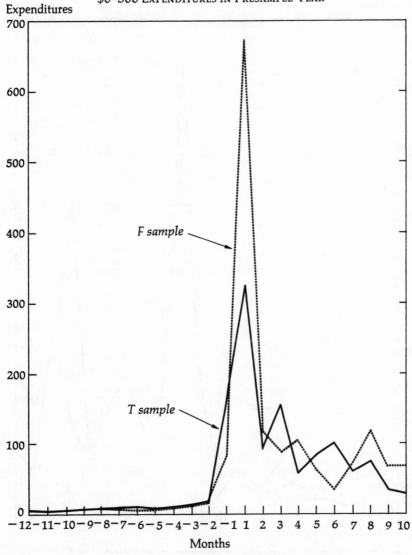

FIGURE 7–3

AVERAGE TOTAL HEALTH CARE EXPENDITURES, PERSONS UNDER SIXTY-FIVE, $300–1,000 EXPENDITURES IN PRESAMPLE YEAR

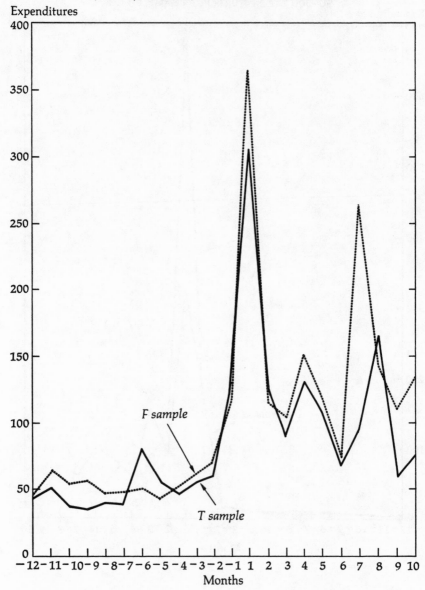

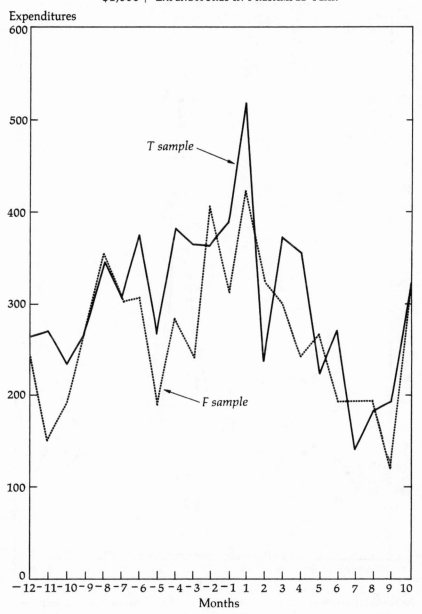

FIGURE 7–4

AVERAGE TOTAL HEALTH CARE EXPENDITURES,
PERSONS UNDER SIXTY-FIVE,
$1,000+ EXPENDITURES IN PRESAMPLE YEAR

Expenditures

T sample

F sample

Months

FIGURE 7–5

Average Total Health Care Expenditures, Persons under Sixty-five

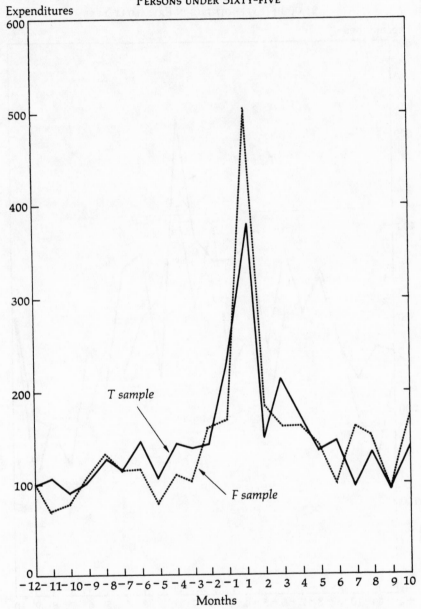

NOTE: Total health care expenditures are obtained from figures 7-2, 7-3, and 7-4 by weighting each group by its proportion in the population: 0.413, 0.260, and 0.327, respectively.

imply afflictions other than duodenal ulcer; expenditures for hospitals and physicians associated with the treatment of duodenal ulcer may be difficult to define or may be recorded less reliably in this case. There is some evidence that this is so: total health care expenditures for the groups with high presample expenditures are in the sample period about the same as, or higher than, those for the groups with lower presample expenditures (table 7–5), but their recorded expenditures for hospitals and physicians associated with diagnoses of duodenal ulcer are about the same (table 7–6).

In spite of the statistically insignificant differences for groups B and C, the differences in overall means for samples T and F are significant for month +1, and for months −1/+1 and −1/+2 as well for expenditures for hospitals and physicians associated with a diagnosis of duodenal ulcer. The significance of these differences may be attributed to the contribution of group A, the fact that the signs of the differences for groups B and C are generally the same as those for group A, and the larger sample that results when the groups are combined. Overall health care expenditures (table 7–5) range from 11 percent less (months −1/+2) to 25 percent less (for month +1). Expenditures for hospitals and physicians associated with a diagnosis of duodenal ulcer are from 40 percent to 63 percent less, days hospitalized from 15 percent to 33 percent less.

An alternative presentation of our findings is provided in table 7–8, where we have controlled for presample health care expenditures by regression on total health care expenditures in the −12/−2 period rather than by stratification. Significant differences between the T and F samples again emerge early in the sample period, most strikingly in the first month. In each case the new technology seems to have the most favorable effect for those patients with the lowest total presample health care expenditures, as shown by comparison of estimated intercepts; for example, total health care expenditures in the first month are $212 less for the T sample ($211) than for the F sample ($423) among patients with no health care expenditures in the presample period. This difference declines as total presample health care expenditures increase and becomes negative when these expenditures exceed $2,700, which is well above the mean expenditure of $1,200. For expenditures for hospitals and physicians associated with the treatment of duodenal ulcer, the break-even point is $25,000, well outside the range of our sample, and for days of hospitalization it is 4.7, which is exceeded only for a few observations in the entire sample.

For later months in the sample period, there are some interesting and significant differences in expenditures between the T and F

TABLE 7–8
COST MEASURES CONTROLLING FOR PRIOR HEALTH CARE EXPENDITURES BY REGRESSION

Dependent Variable[a]	Months	T Sample			F Sample			
		N	Intercept	Slope[b]	N	Intercept	Slope[b]	F[c]
HCE	−1/ +2	500	407 (9.47)	236 (13.2)	633	516 (9.58)	213 (8.65)	1.16
	+1	530	211 (6.33)	106 (7.65)	676	423 (9.33)	27 (1.31)	7.31***
	+2/ +4	395	276 (6.09)	160 (8.71)	533	199 (5.22)	222 (12.6)	3.07**
	+5/ +7	187	203 (3.73)	140 (6.17)	345	205 (5.21)	158 (8.44)	0.30
	+8/+10	51	116 (1.32)	220 (3.90)	136	170 (2.03)	187 (5.92)	0.08
DU HCE	−1/ +2	500	161 (8.13)	−2.56 (0.31)	633	269 (6.64)	−8.28 (0.44)	3.01**
	+1	530	43.1 (5.63)	−1.85 (0.26)	676	266 (6.78)	−10.6 (0.58)	8.52***
	+2/ +4	345	47.5 (4.62)	.080 (0.02)	533	28.3 (3.24)	−.661 (0.16)	1.57

+5/ +7	187	34.4	6.82		345	23.0		−.171		0.94
		(1.86)	(0.88)			(2.00)		(0.03)		
+8/+10	51	.375	−.096		136	14.5		−1.36		0.82
		(1.14)	(0.45)			(1.95)		(0.48)		
DH										
−1/ +2	520	3.98	.634		633	4.52		.260		1.34
		(12.6)	(4.84)			(13.4)		(1.68)		
+1	530	1.73	.266		676	3.62		−.136		14.42***
		(8.15)	(2.94)			(13.6)		(1.10)		
+2/ +4	345	1.87	.380		533	1.25		.478		1.37
		(6.32)	(3.16)			(5.14)		(4.25)		
+5/ +7	187	1.65	.334		345	1.28		.059		2.82*
		(3.69)	(1.82)			(5.92)		(0.60)		
+8/+10	51	1.49	1.08		156	1.09		.075		3.55**
		(1.43)	(1.62)			(2.81)		(0.51)		

NOTE: Ratios of coefficients to standard errors (*t*-statistics) are reported in parentheses. The control variable is total health care expenditures in the −12/−2 period, measured in dollars.

* Significant at the 10 percent level.
** Significant at the 5 percent level.
*** Significant at the 1 percent level.

a. *HCE* denotes total health care expenditures; *DU HCE*, hospital and physician expenditures for duodenal ulcers; *DH*, days hospitalized.

b. Coefficients for *HCE* and *DU HCE* have been scaled by a factor of 1,000.

c. For a test of the hypothesis that intercept and slope coefficients for the T and F samples are the same.

SOURCE: Author.

samples (table 7–8, *HCE* and *DU HCE* dependent variables). In most cases the cimetidine-based technology is relatively more advantageous for patients with low presample expenditures. The only exception worthy of note is total health care expenditures in the +2/+4 period, in which the entire regression and the slope coefficients alone are significantly different and the situation is reversed; the break-even level of presample expenditures here is $1,200. Days hospitalized are directly related to health care expenditures in the presample period for both samples, and the incremental effect is once again greater for the T sample than for the F sample in the periods +5/+7 and +8/+10. In both cases, however, days hospitalized tend to be lower for the F than for the T sample, even when presample health care expenditures are set to zero—that is, the intercept for T is larger than for F. The pattern for days of hospitalization shown in table 7–8 is consistent with the interpretation that the cimetidine technology provides a substitute for surgery in many cases and in some others merely postpones surgery to a later date.

Conclusion

We have set out a method for assessing the effect on total health care expenditures of a change in medical technology, and we have applied the method to a new drug, cimetidine. Federal, state, and local governments are increasingly concerned with rising medical care expenditures, and thus they are often preoccupied with the effect on those expenditures of any change in the health care system, whether it be a change in technology, administrative arrangements, input prices, or anything else. At the same time, as we emphasized in the introduction to this paper, identification of the effect of some activity on expenditures is not generally equivalent to determination of whether it would or would not pass a social benefit-cost test of economic efficiency, let alone a test of its net contribution to social welfare.

In our estimation work we relied on Medicaid records for the state of Texas to determine the expenditure effects of a new drug, cimetidine, recently approved by the Food and Drug Administration for treating duodenal ulcers. Since Medicaid is available largely to the poor, all our data apply to the poor. We are aware of no reason to believe that findings for this population cannot be generalized to the nonpoor population, but we cannot be certain that the two populations are essentially identical in the expenditure effects of the new drug.

TABLE 7–9

Health Care Expenditures, Control Group A, Month +1

	T Sample (N = 149) Mean	Standard deviation	F Sample (N = 206) Mean	Standard deviation	Percentage Reduction, T from F	t-value
Total						
expenditures	325.80	658	663.42	1,406	51	3.02***
Hospital	190.60	520	512.36	1,308	63	3.19***
Physician	80.41	145	117.95	195	32	2.08**
Drugs	29.66	12.9	11.32	8.37	−162	−15.19***
Outpatient	15.80	40.7	15.02	36.5	a	−0.18
Nursing home	4.05	49.4	0.32	4.62	a	−0.91
Other	5.26	17.4	6.43	20.0	a	0.58
Duodenal ulcer						
expenditures	108.63	445	438.32	1,258	75	3.47***
Hospital	84.81	402	404.18	1,225	79	3.49***
Physician	23.81	65.8	34.14	116	a	1.06

** Significant at the 5 percent level.
*** Significant at the 1 percent level.
a. Reduction is statistically insignificant at the 10 percent level.
SOURCE: Author.

We have found that the introduction of cimetidine resulted in a large and statistically significant decrease in expenditures on hospitals and physicians for the treatment of duodenal ulcers for a substantial portion of our sample and smaller but insignificant decreases for the other portion. Whether the new technology is more or less efficacious than the old and whether it has affected morbidity and mortality rates are questions that cannot be addressed using our data base. Whether or not it affects public expenditures for the treatment of this chronic disease over longer periods of time is a question that could be answered with more data of the type used here.

In this study we concentrated on the effect of cimetidine on three broad measures of resources devoted directly to health care: total health care expenditures, expenditures on hospitals and physicians for duodenal ulcers, and days hospitalized. These measures can be disaggregated to provide more detail on the composition of expenditures under the old technology and the new. In tables 7–9 and 7–10, we provide examples of this disaggregation for that part of the

TABLE 7–10

Health Care Expenditures, Control Group A, Months −1/+2

| | T Sample (n = 149) | | F Sample (n = 206) | | Percentage Reduction, | |
	Mean	Standard deviation	Mean	Standard deviation	T from F	t-value
Total						
expenditures	569.76	781	835.22	1,432	32	2.15**
Hospital	336.03	601	602.81	1,322	44	2.45**
Physician	129.68	165	165.41	213	22	1.70*
Drugs	50.50	27.3	23.18	18.3	−118	−10.20***
Outpatient	28.99	54.2	26.97	101	a	−0.23
Nursing home	8.83	104	0.34	4.81	a	−0.95
Other	15.70	47.1	16.47	47.1	a	0.14
Duodenal ulcer						
expenditures	196.95	533	439.26	1,261	55	2.37**
Hospital	164.12	495	402.28	1,242	59	2.39**
Physician	32.83	66.7	36.97	101	a	0.44

* Significant at the 10 percent level.
** Significant at the 5 percent level.
*** Significant at the 1 percent level.
a. Reduction is statistically insignificant at the 10 percent level.
SOURCE: Author.

sample and that period for which differences in the two technologies seem to be the greatest: patients with low presample total health care expenditures in the period immediately surrounding their treatment for duodenal ulcer. Expenditure differentials for the first sample month alone (table 7–9) probably overstate the short-term effect of cimetidine, and those for the last month of the presample and the first two months of the sample period (table 7–10) probably understate it. Whichever estimates are used, however, the same conclusions emerge about the way in which expenditures are reduced by the new technology. The reduction in mean (per capita) total health care expenditures for persons treated with cimetidine—between $265 (table 7–10) and $338 (table 7–9)—is accounted for almost entirely by a reduction in expenditures for hospitals and physicians resulting from the treatment of duodenal ulcer—between $242 and $330. By contrast, the difference in drug costs between the two groups, between $18 and $27, is trivial. This analysis suggests the conjecture that cimetidine has been a substitute for surgery in many cases. If this conjecture

164

is correct, morbidity and mortality due to treatment and the accompanying pain and suffering of patients, relatives, and others are very probably lower in the new technology than in the old. At the same time, we cannot rule out the possibility that use of cimetidine serves primarily to postpone surgery beyond the ten-month sample period covered by this research rather than to eliminate it, although we are aware of no evidence suggesting this outcome.

This new medical care technology, cimetidine, has substitutes in the forms of both surgery and conventional antacids. From the narrow viewpoint of minimizing government expenditure, the question is, Which alternative or combination involves the lowest expenditures? We have not compared all possible treatment combinations, but we have found that using cimetidine does appear to reduce expenditures on treatment of duodenal ulcers compared with the average of other treatment technologies not employing cimetidine.

It would be tempting to conclude that cimetidine is more cost effective than non-cimetidine-using alternatives. It is likely that this is a correct conclusion, subject to two qualifications: (1) longitudinal extension of our data might conceivably show a reversal of the cimetidine therapy's cost advantage, and (2) the efficacy (or, more generally, the benefits) of the various treatment modes and the accompanying health states—morbidity, mortality, pain, and suffering—have not been measured explicitly in our in vivo study (as distinct from a laboratory setting); thus we cannot be certain that the efficacy of the cimetidine technology is at least as great as that of the others.

It seems inappropriate, however, to end on a note of reservation. Regarding point 1, our evidence is that the cost advantage in favor of the cimetidine therapy is not likely to be reversed. Regarding point 2, it seems likely that a therapy that produces a decrease in hospitalization and in medical care expenditures is also bringing about an improvement in the state of patients' health, both because treatment is itself productive of discomfort and disruption of normal work and leisure activities, and because people whose involvement with the medical care system decreases may be presumed to have improved health.

In short, the apparent expenditure-reducing effect of cimetidine therapy, though measuring only average resource *costs*, seems to reflect a favorable *benefit-cost* relationship. In general, a change in expenditures on a commodity is of dubious worth as an index of the net benefits. Reduced expenditures on medical care and specifically on duodenal ulcer therapy, however, reflect both savings in resource costs and increases in social benefits resulting from improved health and decreased demand for medical attention.

Notes

1. A sensitivity analysis of the effects of a number of variables on the present value can be found in Burton A. Weisbrod, "Costs and Benefits of Medical Research: A Case Study of Poliomyelitis," *Journal of Political Economy*, vol. 79 (1971), pp. 527-44; this paper is chapter 5 in the present volume.

2. The nature and therapeutic application of cimetidine cannot be discussed in detail here. For further discussion, see Charles T. Richardson, "Effect of H_2-Receptor Antagonists on Gastric Acid Secretion and Serum Gastrin Concentration," *Gastroenterology*, vol. 74 (November 1978), pp. 366–70; and Daniel H. Winship, "Cimetidine in the Treatment of Duodenal Ulcer," *Gastroenterology*, vol. 74 (November 1978), pp. 402–6.

AUTHOR'S POSTNOTE (December 1982): recently there has developed some evidence of side effects—for example, breast enlargement among males.

3. See Richardson, "Effect of H_2-Receptor Antagonists," and Winship, "Cimetidine in Treatment of Duodenal Ulcer."

4. For a recent attempt to measure these "intangible" effects in the context of a randomized experiment in treating the mentally ill, see chapter 6.

5. Robinson Associates, *The Impact of Cimetidine on the National Cost of Duodenal Ulcers* (Bryn Mawr, Pa.: Robinson Associates, 1978).

6. George von Haunalter and Virginia V. Chandler, *Cost of Ulcer Disease in the United States* (Menlo Park, Calif.: Stanford Research Institute, 1977).

7. Even E_2, however, is subject to shortcomings as a model of reality. In reality, not all duodenal ulcer patients for whom cimetidine is the medically preferred therapy will obtain it—because of misdiagnosis by physicians, failure of the patient to seek medical advice, or failure to heed the advice. Similarly, some patients will actually receive cimetidine even though it is not the medically preferred therapy for their particular set of problems.

8. We might further expect that if the FDA proscription on use of the drug beyond an initial eight-week period reflected the consensus of practitioners, the number of cimetidine prescriptions would eventually decline, as the stock of patients with duodenal ulcers at the time of the drug's introduction was treated once and only those with new ulcers were treated with cimetidine. Certainly there is no evidence that this occurred in the ten months for which we have data (table 7-3), although such a decline might occur beyond the sample period.

8
Concluding Thoughts

Can benefit-cost analysis contribute to improved public policy toward medical research? What are its limitations?

The benefit-cost analyses in the three preceding chapters permit some answers:

1. A benefit-cost analysis undertaken in advance of the expenditure of large amounts of resources on a particular innovation can influence the choice among alternative programs. The benefit-cost evaluation of the Mendota experiment (chapter 6) showed that treating the mentally ill in the community rather than in a hospital can provide substantial benefits in a variety of forms. Although the policy debate continues and no single benefit-cost assessment can hope to be definitive, the analysis can help to narrow the range of issues on which the debate focuses. We found, for example, that the costs of the community-based program were substantial; despite the predictions of both supporters and critics of that approach, however, costs were neither much lower nor much higher than the costs of conventional hospital-based treatment programs.

2. The Mendota study also emphasized what had previously been recognized in the poliomyelitis study (chapter 5): any benefit-cost relationship is an average; as such it is likely to mask the fact that the innovation is probably highly favorable for some population groups—for example, persons with particular mental illness diagnoses or, in the polio vaccine case, young persons—but rather unfavorable for persons with other diagnoses or older persons. Such variation in the benefit-cost relationship among population groups is likely to characterize most social innovations, including medical ones.

3. Even a benefit-cost analysis undertaken after an innovation has been fully implemented can contribute to generalizations about the types of innovations that are most and least likely to pass a benefit-cost test. The evaluation of polio research showed that a medical innovation that prevents disease may entail little cost per person treated but enormous cost per case prevented, since the vast majority

of the population would never have contracted the disease even without the innovation.

4. The current focus of public policy discussions is on soaring expenditures for medical care. The relationship between this focus and a focus on social benefits and costs is seen in the analysis of a new drug to fight duodenal ulcers (chapter 7). Under specified conditions, this study pointed out, an innovation that reduces expenditures would bring about benefits greater than its costs. The study thus suggests that examination of the consequences for expenditures of other medical innovations would sometimes be a useful simplification of a full benefit-cost assessment.

Much more needs to be learned about the social and economic consequences of medical innovations. As the consequences are studied, it is no less important to understand the forces causing such innovations. The growth of medical care insurance, for example, has stimulated not just medical innovations but high-expenditure innovations (chapter 3). The question whether incentives are now stimulating high-cost medical innovations is an important subject for research.

There are many others. To begin with, the notion—implicit in much current thinking—that medical *research* policy can be separated from medical *care* policy is counterproductive if not wrong. Medical research is part of a process that involves not only the expansion of knowledge but also its application. Similarly, evaluation of research is not separable from evaluation of the uses to which its fruits are put. There is no doubt, for example, that the medical research culminating in the Salk and Sabin vaccines against poliomyelitis was successful in producing effective vaccines. Yet their social evaluation hinges on the cost and success of procedures for delivering the vaccines to the population. These depended on pricing policies—by private pharmaceutical firms, physicians, and government agencies—and on policies to let individuals know about the new technology and its effects. The information was disseminated rapidly and at low cost, and poliomyelitis has been virtually eliminated. The new knowledge was successfully applied, and the research that permitted it is estimated to have brought benefits far exceeding costs.

In the mid-1970s the outcome of the swine flu affair was less fortunate. Research had produced a vaccine, but its availability was limited, information regarding its effectiveness was both unclear and poorly disseminated, and serious adverse side effects occurred. At that time the research on the vaccine was unlikely to have passed a social benefit-cost test.[1]

The importance of evaluating any research by its applicability is considerable. This is especially so in the health area because the forces affecting the use of research findings are far from the competitive model: widespread government subsidies (for example, for hospital construction and medical education); private and public health care insurance, which makes it virtually costless for consumers to use new medical technology even though the social cost is high; average-cost pricing practices in hospitals, nursing homes, and other health-care institutions; widespread ignorance among consumers about the quality of health care services; and powerful provider organizations that limit competition—all these combine to make the market for health care, that is, for use of the outcomes of medical research, imperfect. The analyst cannot safely assume, therefore, that the outcomes of medical research will be adopted if and only if they would pass a social benefit-cost test. Socially inefficient technologies may be used because they are profitable given the various price distortions, and socially efficient technologies may go underused or unused for analogous reasons.

The concepts of "socially efficient" and "socially inefficient" are themselves major complications in the evaluation of medical research. To determine whether any particular use of resources is efficient—that is, whether it passes a benefit-cost test—requires placing a value on the medical care and preventive services to which the research gives rise. In most ordinary markets, we are generally willing to value outputs at their observed prices. In health care, by contrast, there is widespread unwillingness to judge value by market prices—partially because of the effects of income inequality on ability to pay and partially because of the price distortions that permeate the medical research and health care industries.

Much of medical research, especially basic research, is financed by the government through the National Institutes of Health. Decisions about which research will be supported are made largely through the peer-review process, in which professional experts judge the quality of proposed research. Although questions have been raised about the limitations of this process, it remains a stronghold where judgments on professional scientific merit dominate political considerations. Yet it is appropriate to ask whether the social desirability of orienting research in one direction or another should be determined solely by researchers. Should society leave it to medical researchers alone to decide how to allocate research resources among problems of the aged and those of infants or youth? Should medical researchers alone decide how to allocate research resources among diseases affecting mortality (such as cancer) and others that affect principally morbidity (such as arthritis)?

What contribution can economic analysis make to the social

process by which such decisions are made? Surely economics—in benefit-cost analysis or any other form—cannot substitute for the technical judgments of scientists. What research scientists can best contribute is judgment about the probabilities of research success along various lines (when undertaken by particular researchers). What they cannot contribute are social valuations of the desirability of various outcomes. In considering the choice between allocating more of a given research budget toward reducing the incidence of some death-causing disease and allocating more toward another disease that causes less mortality but more direct pain and suffering, who should judge the relative importance of saving a life and enhancing the quality of a life by reducing pain? Not medical researchers, I suggest.

Neither, however, have economists any claim to decide such issues. Economic analysis can help: it can show what values people actually place on life-extending versus pain-reducing activities by showing what trade-offs they make; it can clarify the nature of the choices that medical research faces; it can demonstrate that medical research can be subjected to analysis setting forth the kinds of considerations that underlie sound public policy—recognition of the varied forms of costs and benefits, their distribution among population groups, and the consequences of systematic deviation between private and social benefits and costs. Economic analysis, in short, cannot replace medical-scientific judgment. Neither, however, can medical judgment replace economic analysis. In the end, both are vital to the development of sound medical research policy. Yet even together they do not suffice. Society has made it clear that when health and life are at stake, it will not allow access to be rationed by market forces. That low-income persons have more effective demand for health care than they would without government subsidies is well known. What is less-well recognized, though, is that this affects the use of new medical technologies and thus alters incentives to undertake various forms of medical research and development.

Economic analysis in general and benefit-cost analysis in particular can contribute to the development of sound public policy toward medical research. As this book has shown, however, many challenging problems remain. As those who wish to advance the usefulness of benefit-cost analysis in the medical research area work on these problems, it seems well to recognize that such analysis cannot hope to eliminate the need for judgment. It can structure the debate, point up the choices and their implications, and narrow disagreements. But in the end, benefit-cost analysis is an aid to policy formulation—not a substitute for it.

Note

1. For a review and assessment of published economic evaluations of human vaccines, see Burton A. Weisbrod and John Huston, "Benefits and Costs of Vaccines: An Evaluative Survey," University of Wisconsin-Madison, Department of Economics, February 1983.

A NOTE ON THE BOOK

This book was edited by Donna Spitler
and by Claire Theune of the
Publications Staff of the American Enterprise Institute.
The staff also designed the cover and format, with Pat Taylor.
The figures were drawn by Hördur Karlsson.
The text was set in Palatino, a typeface designed by Hermann Zapf.
Hendricks-Miller Typographic Company, of Washington, D.C.,
set the type, and BookCrafters of Chelsea, Michigan, printed and
bound the book, using paper made by the P. H. Glatfelter Company.